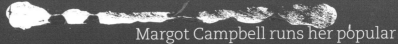

Margot Campbell runs her popular
Pilates on the go… studio in West
London. Working with people of all
ages and shapes, Margot has adapted
her methods to help her clients
achieve their goals, whatever their
schedule. Margot has worked with a
number of high profile clients over
the years.

To mum, dad and gordon…
better late than never! x

Margot Campbell
Pilates on the go

HODDER &
STOUGHTON

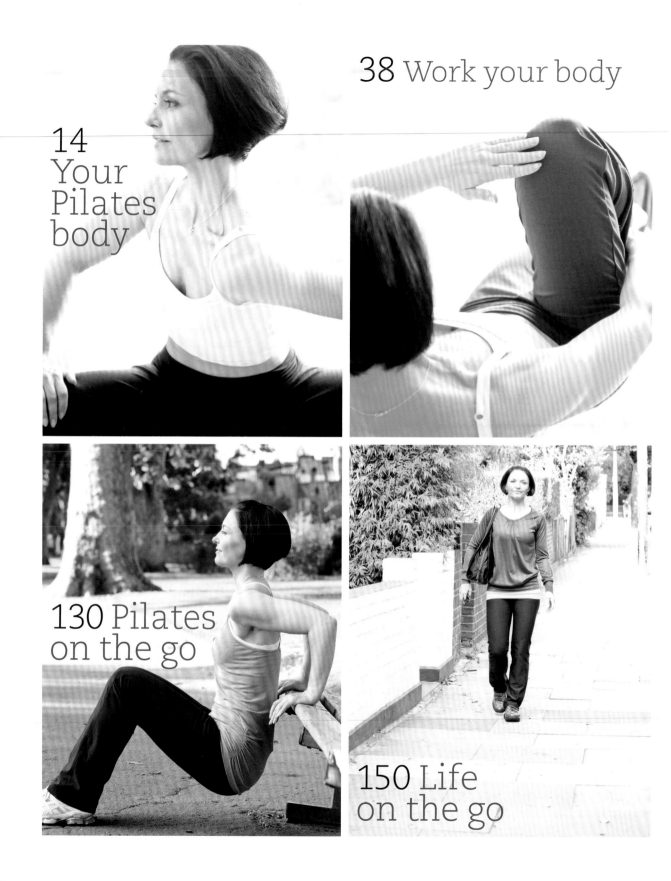

Contents

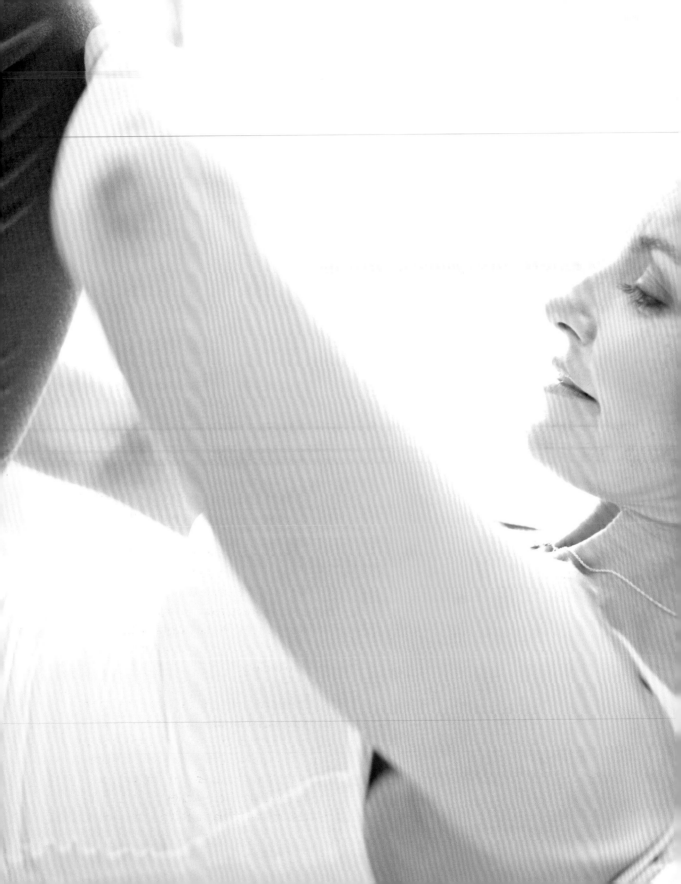

Introduction – change your body shape

Welcome to Pilates on the go. At my studio in West London, I work with people individually and in small groups and this is the programme I have devised over many years of teaching Pilates that works so well for all my clients. But obviously not everyone can make it to a class and there's no reason why you can't follow my programme at home which is why I've decided to write this book.

Over the years I've been lucky enough to work with all sorts of people, some well known and others not, but regardless of who they are if the client is prepared to commit to the programme, I've seen bodies change shape and attitudes transform as they embrace this holistic, incredibly effective body and mind fitness plan. And I promise the same can happen for you.

If you want your body to feel toned and look even better, you've come to the right place. If you'd like to focus on a trouble area, such as your arms, your abdominals (abs) or your bottom, you'll love my targeted workouts. They'll knock years off your appearance in just a few short weeks. And if all you desire is to drop a dress size or two, I've even put together diet, lifestyle and exercise plans so that you can enjoy happy and healthy weight loss and get fit all at the same time.

The beauty of Pilates is that you lengthen, strengthen and tone your body without building muscle bulk. So you become lean and toned – a pretty great combination. Your flexibility will also improve, as will lifestyle-related niggles, such as stiff shoulders. Once your core (your tummy area) has strengthened, you will feel more grounded and at one with your body. You'll walk with easy grace and poise, your improved posture will take inches off your waistline and even your breathing will improve, giving you more energy and relaxing your mind.

This book is a total body and mind workout, so in addition to the core Pilates exercises I have included some cardio exercises that will raise your heart rate, plus a lifestyle plan that encompasses diet, tips for doing Pilates exercises throughout the day (yes, you can definitely work your arms while you wait for the kettle to boil!) and how to relieve physical signs of stress. Suggestions to help you stay fit and flexible while working or looking after small children are also included.

We start in exactly the same way as I start with my new clients – by filling in a simple but very helpful questionnaire. From this, you will soon see exactly what your goals are and what you need to do to achieve them. I will also help you get to know your own body – what parts of it do you like,

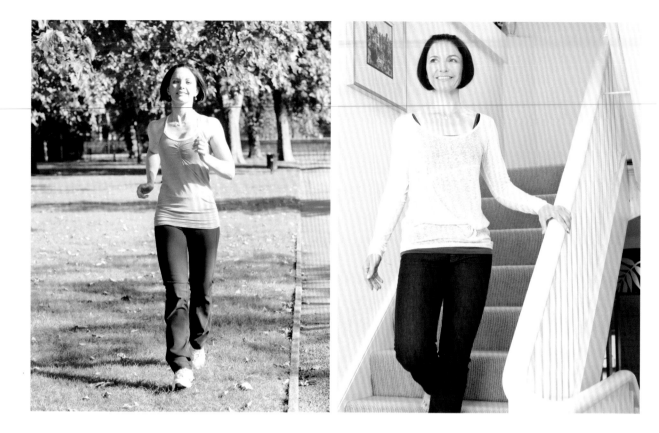

what would you like to improve. And very early on, we look at how you walk, sit and stand. By making just a few small adjustments in these areas, you will start to look and feel better straightaway.

I first became interested in Pilates when I was looking for a different form of fitness. I was a keen runner and enjoyed many aerobics classes but I was looking for something that had a calming and relaxing aspect to it that I could fit into my busy lifestyle. I felt that life was becoming a bit too hectic and wanted to feel more balanced again.

I discovered that, with Pilates, you work on your body's strength and flexibility but at a calmer, more relaxed pace than in the

classes I was used to. I felt I was able to get to know my body more thoroughly in this way – where my strengths and weaknesses lay and how to feel centred and relaxed – while the tone in my muscles improved beyond belief. Everything started to defy gravity!

The best thing about Pilates is that once you pick it up, it really gives results because you can work it into your daily life. As you walk, you will be able to draw in and tone your tummy gently. You'll look after your back as you lift objects (and small children!) and you'll be able to incorporate some of the exercises into your day, even while sitting at your desk. You'll also feel in relaxed control of your body and be more resilient to the stresses of everyday life, and furthermore it will just make you feel

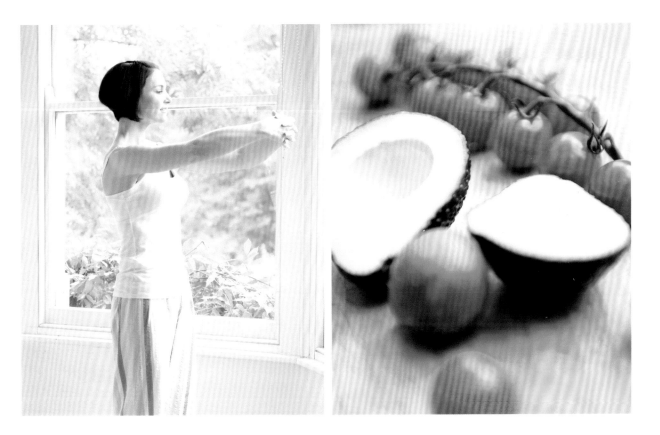

good. So whether you're a complete beginner, top athlete, housewife or busy executive, Pilates really can make a difference in helping you to tone and reshape your body.

Making a positive change, such as taking up this programme, tends to have a positive effect on your lifestyle in general, and that's when you will see the most dramatic results. I encourage you, as I do all my clients, to think where you can fit in little bursts of exercise throughout the day, from stepping up your walking pace to doing a few bottom exercises during the ad breaks of your favourite television programmes. I've even created a 5 Minutes in the Morning routine that you can simply roll out of bed and do first thing.

I have exactly the same philosophy when it comes to a healthy diet. I'm not going to give you a long list of what not to eat, but rather I hope you'll want to add plenty of light, fresh healthy foods to your day as you begin to take care of your body. There are 14 days of menu plans to get you started and give you lots of ideas, plus a mini cellulite-busting plan!

Put it all together and you will be amazed at the results. Always dreamed of defined arms? Wish you could have a pert bottom? Wishing away your post-baby tummy? These are all goals that you can reach with a good dose of motivation combined with exercises that really do work. So, it's probably about time we got you started!

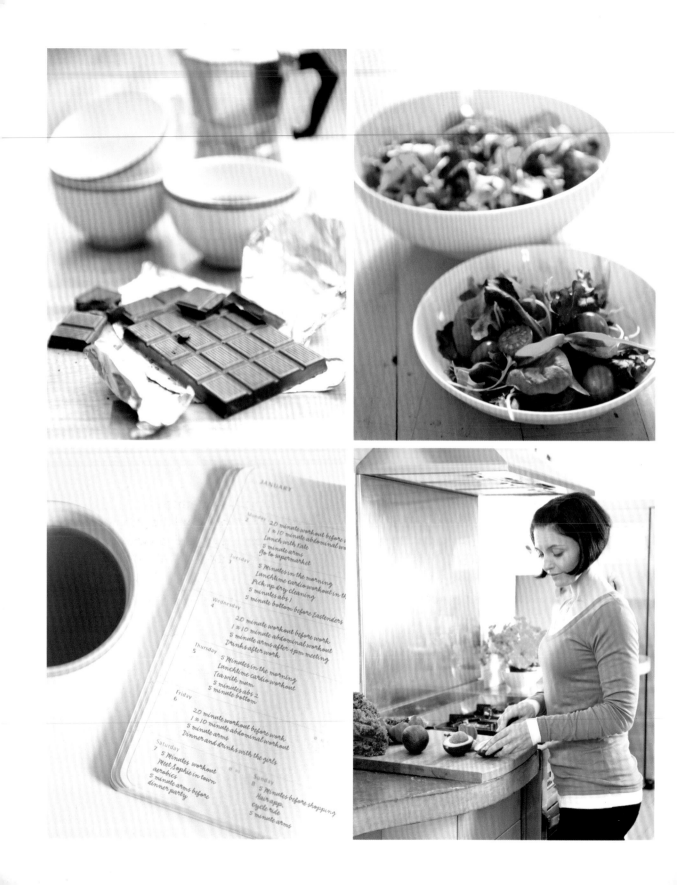

Questionnaire

Whenever I meet a new client, I ask a few quick questions the answers to which help me create the perfect plan for that individual, based on their own goals and just how much effort they are happy to put in. The key with any change in lifestyle or new exercise programme is to take it at a pace that certainly pushes you a little but that you can embrace, rather than trying too much too soon and giving up almost before you've started.

What's your starting point?

How many times do you exercise for at least 30 minutes during an average week? The answer to this question gives a good indication of your current level of fitness.

Please don't worry if the answer to this question is along the lines of 'er, zero'. That just means you will improve right from the beginning. Exercise really is for everyone – the key is to take it at a pace that is right for you. The routines in this book will work together to boost your general fitness while starting to give your body some tone and definition. So if running up the stairs leaves you feeling out of puff, prepare to add a little fitness to your life and reap the benefits.

If you answered 2–3 times a week, you have already made a good start with your fitness but perhaps you realise that walking round the park isn't quite going to cut it if you want that perfect bum! Maybe you'd like to try something new and put a bit more effort into your fitness to get to the next level.

If your answer was in the realms of 4–7 times a week, it's a good bet that you are already fit but perhaps want to add a few new ideas to your repertoire, or you'd like to focus on toning up your body shape, either all over or a specific target area.

What do you want to achieve?

* Would you like to improve your general health and fitness?
* Would you like to lose weight?
* Would you like the perfect bum/flat tummy/defined arms?
* Would you like all of the above?

If you've picked up this book to take a positive step in the right direction in terms of your health and fitness, you are going to love all of the Target Zone workouts, and I hope you'll be making the 5 Minutes in the Morning routine part of your daily ritual. I've also included cardio workouts for the home and park so that you can sculpt your body through the Pilates routines and also improve your aerobic fitness.

If you're keen to lose weight, the great news is that by adding exercise to a healthy eating plan you will make it so much easier to drop those extra pounds. Plus, you're much more likely to keep the weight off in the long run because you'll have boosted your metabolism and developed an active,

healthy lifestyle. Active people tend to be more energised and stay slim without having to carry a calorie calculator and say 'no thanks' every time a box of chocolates is passed around!

If you'd like to target a particular area of your body, try the workouts that I've designed to focus on three main zones – abs; back, arms and chest; bottom and thighs. You'll still work your whole body but you can emphasise those particular areas in your weekly plan. So if you want 'that bum', or if you'd dearly love to tone up your underarms, and have the odd spare five minutes in your day, you can do a few squats (best exercise in the world for bottoms) or grab your band for some quick arm exercises.

Have you thought about what you eat?

* Are you happy with your weight?
* Are you happy with your diet?

Exercise alone can't answer all weight-loss prayers. It can make weight much easier to lose, but you need to combine it with healthy eating. Fortunately, one tends to encourage the other – a banana gives you a much better energy boost before a workout than a chocolate bar or a packet of biscuits. If you already have a fantastically healthy diet but struggle to lose weight, upping your exercise may just make the difference.

I encourage everyone to take a gentle look at their portions – simply eating a little less during the day will help you achieve the results you want.

I have included a section on healthy eating plus two weeks of menus to go alongside the exercise plans. By putting the diet and exercise together, you'll drop pounds as well as inches!

What about your lifestyle?

* Do you lead a very busy, stressful life?
* Do you burn the candle at both ends, or wish you could find just a few more hours in the day for some 'me time'?

Life is a juggling act nowadays. Clients often ask me how they can make their days more active without having to turn their lives upside down; trying to find the time. The trick is to use this book and programme as a real boost in motivation to take care of your fitness and your general health and wellbeing. After all, if you are feeling fit and healthy, you'll have tons more energy and be able to get so much more done in the day!

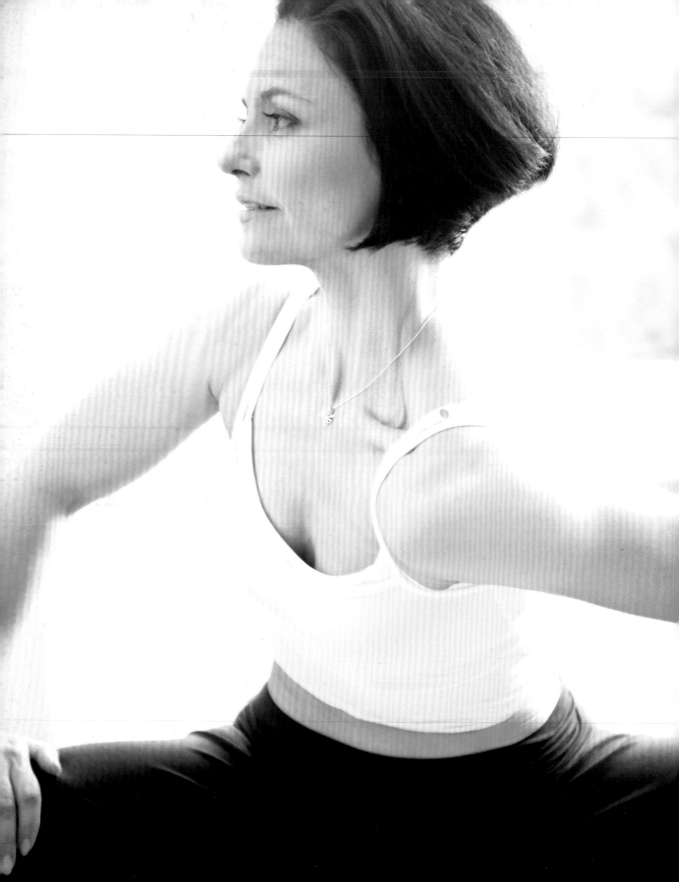

Your Pilates body

Why Pilates?

I fell in love with Pilates because it is a unique form of exercise that not only conditions and tones the body but is also wonderfully relaxing for the mind. Pilates makes you lean, strong and flexible, which is why it's so good for problem areas such as stomachs, bottoms, arms and thighs. That's why women love Pilates. For many top professional sportsmen, the attraction is the way Pilates builds core strength and works muscles without compromising agility and speed.

Pilates is also an increasingly popular exercise as a form of physiotherapy. For example, many people recovering from hip surgery or with problem backs find that working one-to-one with an experienced Pilates teacher can be greatly beneficial.

Pilates was developed in Germany about a century ago by Joseph H. Pilates, first as a way to strengthen his own body after suffering with asthma and rickets as a child, then to help prison camp internees keep up their strength during the First World War. In 1926 Joseph Pilates set up his first studio in New York, the spiritual home of Pilates. Broadway dancers were among the first fans. The exercises helped them look slim and lean while they developed strength and amazing body control.

Today, Pilates is just as popular as ever. In my studio, I combine classic Pilates moves with a few modified exercises to give you exactly the results you desire. So while this book isn't a 'classic' Pilates bible, I hope

'Margot's techniques have transformed my posture and my body, plus they energise and motivate me to be more active throughout the day. I work as an advertising executive and used to let my fitness fly out of the window at the first sign of stress but now I know how I can fit exercise into my life easily, and as something I really look forward to. I don't think I could imagine life without Pilates now!' Caroline

you'll love these routines as much as my clients do, and enjoy equally positive results. I teach such a wide range of people from all walks of life. People with very busy lives love the calm feeling that comes over them while they also happen to be giving their body a really good workout. Sports people and dancers love the sense of control Pilates gives them while keeping them agile and light on their feet. Models adore the body definition that comes with Pilates, which for women is both feminine and strong, the perfect combination. I have clients who come to me during pregnancy and also afterwards to get back into shape. These exercises really can be enjoyed by anyone at any age.

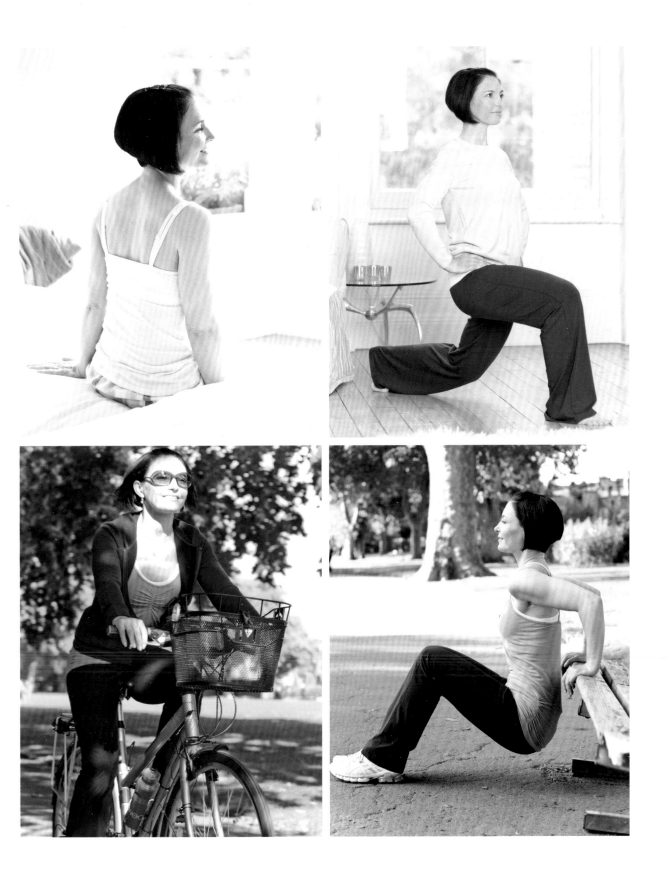

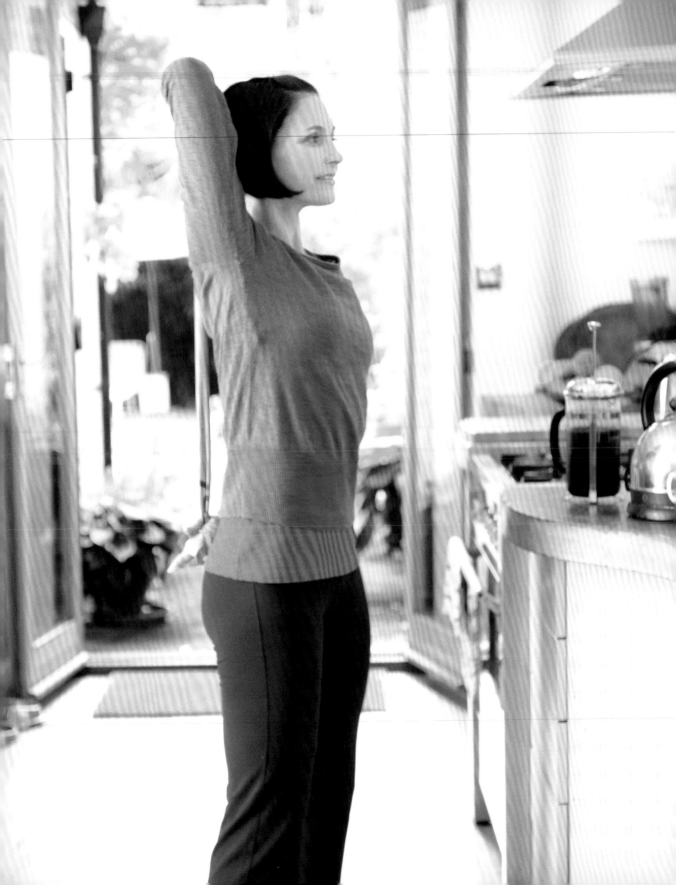

The workouts explained

To keep your interest, motivation and therefore your energy levels high, a really good class or workout won't be exactly the same from one week to the next. That's why I have included plenty of variety in the workouts in this book. So when planning your exercise for the week, mix things up a bit and create a plan that really works for you.

Target Zone Workouts

– Abdominals

– Back, arms and chest

– Bottom and thighs

Each of these workouts focuses on a specific area while also improving your overall body tone and fitness. Each one takes approximately 10 minutes to complete.

20 Minute Workout

This brings together a taste of all three of the Target Zones for a fantastic, quick and intense workout.

5 Minute Workouts

I have created these to fit into your day when you have just a few minutes to spare. The 5 Minute Morning workout is a lovely stretch and wake-up routine – you can roll out of bed and do it in your pyjamas. Put the kettle on, grab your band and do 5 Minute Arms, and if you want a perfect bottom, jump up during the ad breaks for a few squats and lunges from the 5 Minute Bottom and Thighs workout and you'll soon see the difference.

What equipment do you need?

∗ Mat

∗ Exercise band

∗ An outfit that makes you feel fab

∗ Trainers

∗ Water bottle

A nice excuse to go shopping!

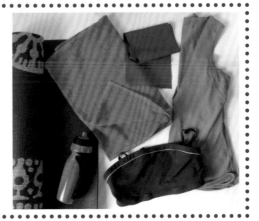

Home and Park Cardio Workouts

Cardio exercise simply means exercise that raises your heart rate, such as cycling, jogging or skipping. Add the exercises I recommend to your weekly routine and you will speed up the results you see and feel in your body. Not only will working out in short bursts burn calories during and even after you exercise, but this kind of exercise will really get your endorphins flowing quickly so that you feel the natural high that follows a good workout session.

Short bursts of cardio exercise are an essential part of the personal fitness plans I develop for my clients. So while clients may come to the studio just once a week, there is plenty they can do on the other days to boost their fitness and keep the pounds falling off. Therefore I encourage everyone to include a couple of 15 minute Home or Park Cardio workouts in their exercise plan, plus a couple of different fitness activities e.g. swimming, tennis or even an aerobics class, when they have some free time. In addition, any Cardio on the go activities you can incorporate into your day e.g. taking the stairs while at work or doing a few Squats or Star Jumps during TV intermissions, will all add up.

'I've just never been able to convince myself to go to the gym on a regular basis. All those machines and fit people. I never even liked netball at school! But the beauty of Pilates, I have found, is that you can go completely at your own pace and whatever your starting point, you simply improve from there. I was an absolute novice when I started, but once I grasped the basics of breathing and drawing in your connection I realised that so long as I was working as hard as I could, I began improving literally from that first day. Pilates really is for anyone, whether a sports fanatic or for people like me who want to bring some exercise into their life for the first time.' Kate

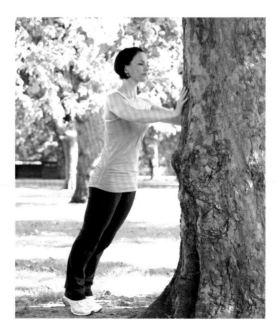

Putting it all together

* Enjoy a low-fat latte or a cup of tea and some 'me time' while you devise your plan to change your body shape. You'll need to call on all your motivation, so be realistic and don't impose unfair expectations on yourself. Set goals that you can make happen.

* Say you really want to improve the tone and shape of your body, build up your cardio fitness and get a flatter stomach, you might slot in three 20 Minute Workouts, two 15 Minute Home or Park Cardio Workouts and three 10 Minute Abdominal Workouts, plus a couple of fitness activities at the weekend e.g. an aerobics class or cycle ride.

* At the end of each week, take a bit of time to focus on everything you have achieved, from the routines you have completed to all the delicious healthy food you have been eating. Don't beat yourself up if you haven't achieved everything you set out for the week. Just keep moving forward – there's always tomorrow!

* Download your favourite tracks on to your mp3 player, iPod or whatever system you have, to help you along on your workouts – even doing the housework with the stereo on is a great motivator – and always remember to warm up and cool down.

* Fit in the 5 Minute routines, or a couple of Cardio on the go activities, while you wait for the kettle to boil, watch television or just have a few minutes to spare. We're all creatures of habit, so if you can create some healthy practices that begin to fit naturally into your day, not only will you change your body shape but this way of living will last a lifetime. Prepare to become a 'fittie'!

Exercise menu

* 10 Minute Abs
* 10 Minute Back, Arms and Chest
* 10 Minute Bottom and Thighs
* 20 Minute Workout
* 5 Minutes in the Morning
* 5 Minute Abs/Arms/Bottom and Thighs
* 15 Minute Home and Park Cardio Workouts

On the following pages you'll find a 14-day plan I've put together, picked from the work-outs on the menu. I've also suggested some healthy food options (see pages 28–33) to help you plan your first couple of weeks – all you need to get started on the new you!

14 days at a glance
Exercise: *Week one*

Monday

* 20 Minute Workout
* 1 x 10 Minute Abdominal Workout
* 5 Minute Arms

Tuesday

* 5 Minutes in the Morning
* Home/Park Cardio Workout
* 5 Minutes Abs 1
* 5 Minute Bottom and Thighs

Wednesday

* 20 Minute Workout
* 1 x 10 Minute Abdominal Workout
* 5 Minute Arms

Thursday

* 5 Minutes in the Morning
* Home/Park Cardio Workout
* 5 Minutes Abs 2
* 5 Minute Bottom and Thighs

Friday

* 20 Minute Workout
* 1 x 10 Minute Abdominal Workout
* 5 Minute Arms

Saturday

* 5 Minutes in the Morning
* Fitness activity (aerobics)
* 5 Minute Arms

Sunday

* 5 Minutes in the Morning
* Fitness activity (cycle ride)
* 5 Minute Arms

**Monday
2**

20 minute workout before work
1 x 10 minute abdominal workout
Lunch with Kate
5 minute arms
Go to supermarket

**Tuesday
3**

5 Minutes in the morning
Lunchtime cardio workout in the park
Pick up dry cleaning
5 minutes abs 1
5 minute bottom before Eastenders

**Wednesday
4**

20 minute workout before work
1 x 10 minute abdominal workout
5 minute arms after 4pm meeting
Drinks after work

**Thursday
5**

5 Minutes in the morning
Lunchtime cardio workout
Tea with mum
5 minutes abs 2
5 minute bottom

**Friday
6**

20 minute workout before work
1 x 10 minute abdominal workout
5 minute arms
Dinner and drinks with the girls

**Saturday
7**

5 Minutes workout
Meet Sophie in town
aerobics
5 minute arms before
dinner party

**Sunday
8**

5 Minutes before shopping
Hair app.
cycle ride
5 minute arms

Exercise: *Week two*

Monday

* 20 Minute Workout
* 1 x 10 Minute Abdominal Workout
* 5 Minute Arms

Tuesday

* 5 Minutes in the Morning
* Home/Park Cardio Workout
* 5 Minutes Abs 1
* 5 Minute Bottom and Thighs

Wednesday

* 20 Minute Workout
* 1 x 10 Minute Abdominal Workout
* 5 Minute Arms

Thursday

* 5 Minutes in the Morning
* Home/Park Cardio Workout
* 5 Minutes Abs 2
* 5 Minute Bottom and Thighs

Friday

* 20 Minute Workout
* 1 x 10 Minute Abdominal Workout
* 5 Minute Arms

Saturday

* 5 Minutes in the Morning
* Fitness activity (aerobics)
* 5 Minute Arms

Sunday

* 5 Minutes in the Morning
* Fitness activity (cycle ride)
* 5 Minute Arms

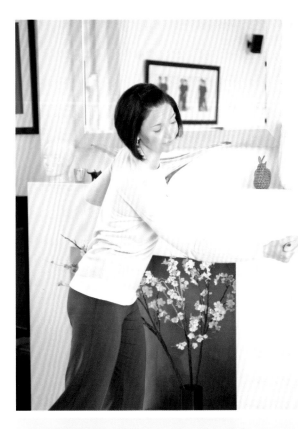

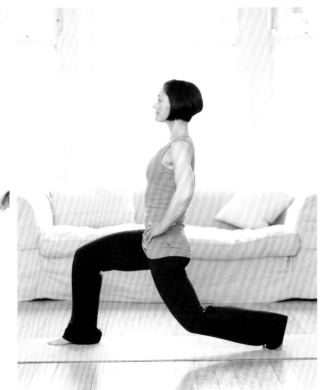

Fitness activities

These are a few examples of fitness activities you can try to incorporate into your exercise plan when you have some time to spare.

∗ Swimming: try one length of front crawl, followed by one length of breaststroke and one of backstroke, and one using a float to support your hands so that you use just your legs. Then try putting the float between the thighs and using just your arms

∗ Cycling trip followed by afternoon tea

∗ Play Frisbee with the children

∗ Game of tennis, squash or badminton

∗ An aerobics class

∗ Sign up for that 5K challenge – you know you want to!

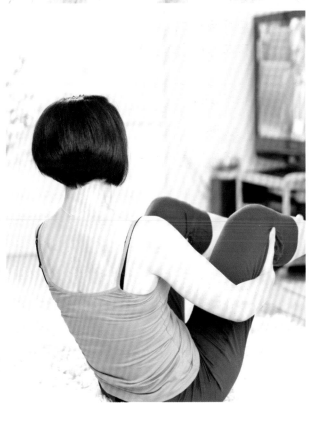

Diet on the go

So what's on the menu? I am no diet guru but as someone who cares about my body and my health I have a balanced approach to eating that works for my busy lifestyle. I know that being healthy on the inside is as important as being healthy on the outside, so have a think about what you eat. We all should be aiming for a balanced diet, not too much of one food group or too little of another. The trick is to aim for a diet with everything in moderation.

Think fresh, seasonal, colourful and natural.

Planning your meals in advance, taking your lunch to work so you're not tempted by calorie-laden sandwiches and crisps, and writing both your exercise plan and diet diary are all changes that will make a big difference to your overall health and waistline. The best thing about doubling up fitness with healthy eating is that you get double the results, and they last.

Margot's top 10 steps to healthy eating

1 Eat a good breakfast, have a morning snack, try to make lunch your main meal of the day, have an afternoon snack and evening meal.

2 Eating little and often will keep your blood sugar nicely balanced and your energy levels sustained throughout the day.

3 Keep food simple, seasonal, light, fresh and colourful.

4 Bear in mind size of portions – think moderation!

5 Always try to eat sitting down and eat slowly to aid your digestion. Take some time out to enjoy your food.

6 Skip the faddy diets – they almost always make you want to scream or eat a tub of ice cream in one sitting when you fall off the wagon!

7 Replace ready meals with light and simple home-cooked suppers. Treat yourself to a new cookbook or two and get adventurous in the kitchen.

8 Small changes will be much more likely to last than big ones, especially when teamed up with exercise.

9 Keep hydrated throughout the day by drinking plenty of still water and your favourite herbal teas.

10 Replace some of your sweet treats with other ways to be nice to yourself, such as taking a long, luxurious bath or curling up with your favourite book. The odd slice of cake won't do you any harm, but just always think moderation!

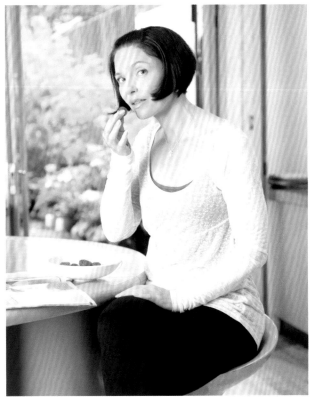

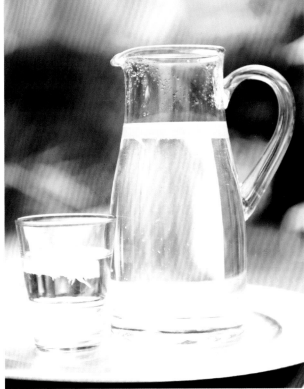

Fuel your workouts

Choose wholegrains for slow energy release and lean protein (chicken and fish) for power, and eat plenty of fruits and vegetables throughout the day.

Before a workout, a banana or cereal is perfect, and afterwards make sure to eat some protein to help your muscles recover quickly – just in time for another workout tomorrow!

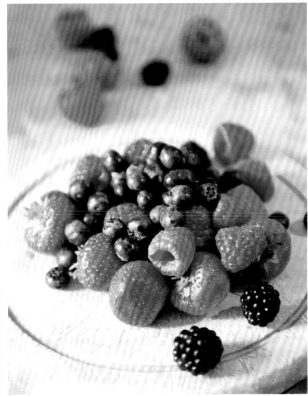

Your shopping list

Fresh and seasonal

Fruit: apples, apricots, bananas, blackberries, blueberries, cherries, clementines, figs, grapefruit, grapes, lemons, limes, mangoes, melon, oranges, peaches, plums, pears, pineapple, raspberries, strawberries

Vegetables: asparagus, avocados, baby spinach leaves, bean sprouts, beetroot, broccoli, butternut squash, carrots, celery, courgettes, cucumber, fennel, green beans, leeks, lettuce leaves, mange tout, mushrooms, onions (red, white and spring), peppers, potatoes (new and small jackets), rocket, sweet corn (on the cob), tomatoes

Herbs: basil, coriander, garlic, ginger, mint, parsley, rosemary, thyme

Chilled

Cottage cheese with pineapple
Frozen peas
Hummus
Light cream cheese
Natural or Greek yoghurt (regular or fat free)
Parmesan cheese
Semi-skimmed milk
Soups
Yakult

Meat and fish

Chicken breasts
Cod fillets
Cooked prawns
Parma ham
Pork medallions
Salmon fillets
Sardines
Smoked mackerel fillets
Smoked salmon
Steaks

Bakery and cereals

Muesli (no added sugar)
Porridge oats
Wholegrain, rye or sourdough bread

Grocery

Baked beans
Balsamic vinegar
Black pepper
Brown rice
Canned mixed beans
Canned tomatoes
Canned tuna in spring water
Chilli paste
Couscous
Dark chocolate
Dijon mustard
Dried fruit (apricots, figs, prunes, sultanas)
Dried herbs and spices
Eggs
Egg noodles
Extra virgin olive oil
Harissa paste
Herbal teas
Honey
Lemon juice
Mayonnaise (low fat)
Nuts – almonds, hazelnuts, mixed
Oatcakes
Peanut butter
Sea salt
Seeds – mixed, pumpkin, sunflower
Soy sauce
Stocks – chicken and vegetable
Tomato puree

Eating out tips

✳ Go for simple dishes that have been steamed, grilled or poached, avoiding anything fried or battered.

✳ Choose sauces that are tomato based rather than creamy or cheesy.

✳ Consider a starter and a couple of vegetable side dishes as your main course.

✳ Ask your waiter for the healthiest, most delicious recommendations.

✳ Ignore the bread basket, and if you do arrive hungry, order a spicy tomato juice to keep you going.

14 days at a glance
Diet: *Week one*

Monday

Breakfast: porridge with blueberries and a drizzle of honey

Snack: pear and a small handful of almonds

Lunch: chicken, avocado and rocket wrap with a squeeze of lemon juice

Snack: small pot of natural yoghurt and berries

Dinner: vegetable stir-fry with a small portion of egg noodles

Tuesday

Breakfast: 2 slices of wholemeal toast spread with peanut butter

Snack: small punnet of blueberries and a small handful of pumpkin seeds

Lunch: tuna salad with 3 smallish new potatoes, green beans, mixed leaves, salad onions and balsamic vinegar

Snack: cottage cheese and pineapple

Dinner: mushroom omelette (2 eggs) with tomatoes and basil

Friday

Breakfast: soft boiled egg and soldiers

Snack: small pot of natural yoghurt and berries

Lunch: carrot and coriander soup with chicken and avocado wholemeal wrap

Snack: 2 dried apricots and a small handful of mixed nuts

Dinner: minute steak with sautéed onions, courgettes and mixed peppers, and a light sauce of honey and Dijon mustard

Saturday

Breakfast: grilled mushrooms and tomatoes on wholemeal or rye toast

Snack: banana

Lunch: grilled fillet of cod with harissa-paste rub, 3 smallish new potatoes and braised fennel

Snack: strip of dark chocolate (about 20g) and a handful of mixed nuts

Dinner: speedy stir-fry of prawns, mange tout, courgettes, carrots, peppers, beansprouts, chilli paste and lemon juice

Wednesday

Breakfast: porridge with soft dried prunes and a drizzle of honey

Snack: 2 oatcakes with hummus

Lunch: grilled chicken with green beans, mixed leaves, a dressing of extra virgin olive oil and lemon juice, and a slice of crusty bread

Snack: banana

Dinner: carrot and coriander soup, wholemeal wrap with light cream cheese and cucumber

Thursday

Breakfast: small bowl of muesli with semi-skimmed milk or natural yoghurt and raspberries

Snack: 2 clementines or an apple

Lunch: smoked mackerel fillet with ½ an avocado and mixed salad with a squeeze of lemon juice and a little extra virgin olive oil

Snack: about 20 grapes and a small handful of almonds

Dinner: beans on 2 slices of wholemeal toast

Sunday

Breakfast: scrambled eggs with smoked salmon

Snack: small punnet of blueberries and a small handful of pumpkin seeds

Lunch: lemon and honey roast chicken with roast carrots, red onion, butternut squash and steamed broccoli (make extra roasted veg for soup)

Snack: slice of wholemeal toast spread with peanut butter

Dinner: steamed asparagus with Parma ham and balsamic dressing

Drinks

∗ Keep hydrated by drinking water throughout the day, especially before, during and after your workouts. This will keep you energised, plus water is fabulous for your skin and for reducing bloating around your middle, so you can really show off your newly toned waist.

∗ I like to have a juice drink once a day. I love the combination of freshly squeezed orange, beetroot, apple, celery and ginger, but I must admit you do have to like beetroot! Why not experiment with the fruits and veg you particularly like?

∗ I also have a little bottle of a yoghurt drink, each day. It's my daily dose of good bacteria, which helps maintain and support a healthy digestive system.

Diet: *Week two*

Monday

Breakfast: porridge with raspberries and a drizzle of honey

Snack: 2 dried apricots and a small handful of almonds

Lunch: leftover cold roast chicken with salad leaves, ½ an avocado with a dressing of extra virgin olive oil and lemon juice

Snack: 2 oatcakes with hummus and carrot sticks

Dinner: roasted vegetable soup with crusty wholemeal bread. To make the soup, heat veg in a pan with chicken stock and fresh thyme, and whiz in a blender until smooth

Tuesday

Breakfast: soft boiled egg and soldiers

Snack: apple or 2 clementines

Lunch: prawn salad

Snack: banana

Dinner: pea and mint soup with a slice of crusty wholemeal bread. To make the soup, sauté a chopped onion in a little olive oil; add 400ml vegetable or chicken stock and bring to the boil; add a 480g packet of frozen peas and simmer for five minutes; add torn fresh mint, seasoning and blitz in a blender

Friday

Breakfast: 2 slices of wholemeal toast spread with peanut butter

Snack: small pot of natural yoghurt with berries

Lunch: rest of Italian bean soup with a wholemeal wrap

Snack: strip of dark chocolate and some blueberries

Dinner: grilled salmon with grated ginger and lime juice, and a cucumber and green salad dressed with lime, basil and vinegar

Saturday

Breakfast: fruit salad of grapefruit, orange, Greek yoghurt and honey

Snack: 2 dried apricots and a handful of mixed seeds

Lunch: butternut squash soup with cucumber and light cream cheese wholemeal wrap

Snack: hummus and crudités

Dinner: grilled sardines (2 large or 3 small) with green beans and tomato and onion salad dressed with basil, lemon juice and extra virgin olive oil

Try to make lunch your main meal of the day and go for smaller portions in the evening.

Wednesday

Breakfast: muesli with sliced banana and semi-skimmed milk

Snack: small punnet of blueberries and a handful of pumpkin seeds

Lunch: roasted peppers stuffed with goat's cheese, pine nuts, cherry tomatoes (halved) and chopped basil

Snack: slice of wholemeal toast spread with peanut butter

Dinner: corn on the cob with a little butter and lots of black pepper; baked apple stuffed with sultanas and a drizzle of honey

Thursday

Breakfast: porridge with prunes and a drizzle of honey

Snack: 2 oatcakes with hummus

Lunch: tuna salad with 3 smallish new potatoes, green beans, mixed leaves, salad onions and balsamic dressing

Snack: about 20 grapes and a small handful of almonds

Dinner: Italian bean soup. To make it, heat up some chicken stock, a can of mixed beans, crushed garlic, some tomato puree and chopped parsley. Sprinkle with a little Parmesan cheese before serving

Sunday

Breakfast: scrambled eggs with sautéed mushrooms on a slice of whole-meal toast

Snack: pear and a small handful of almonds

Lunch: medallions of pork loin with sautéed leeks, carrots and a small jacket potato

Snack: strip of dark chocolate and some strawberries

Dinner: Parma ham, fig and rocket salad with balsamic dressing

Drinks

∗ Hot water and lemon is a fabulously refreshing way to start the day.

∗ My favourite herbal teas are peppermint, and ginger and lemon. Herbal teas will boost your fluid intake for the day and often promote good digestion, general health and wellbeing, or are simply relaxing. Chamomile is one of those. Great while I'm working in the studio.

∗ Alcohol – to have or not to have? A little bit of what you fancy won't do you any harm, and denying yourself may result in over-indulgence when you do finally allow yourself to partake! Just think moderation!

CELLULITE

The leg, bottom and thigh exercises in the workouts will soon have cellulite running for the hills, and you can help it on its way by eating a few more cellulite-busting foods and a few less of the foods that tend to make cellulite more prominent. The dimple-like appearance of cellulite can be caused by a less than clean diet, which is why I always recommend going for as many fresh and natural foods as you possibly can, meaning foods that are as close to their natural appearance as possible. So, for example, it's always better to have boiled new potatoes rather than crisps or chips.

* Fruit and veg in particular contain antioxidants, which help to remove toxins from the body and therefore help skin's natural elasticity.

* Berries are excellent because they contain such high levels of antioxidants. Add a handful to your morning muesli or porridge, and snack on them throughout the day. They are high in vitamin C, which is thought to boost levels of collagen in the skin for a firmer appearance, and are naturally sweet but contain very few calories. They are definitely on my own list of 'super' foods.

* The essential fatty acids found in oily fish such as salmon, mackerel, tuna and sardines are excellent for improving the skin's natural radiance and so help your complexion.

* Natural 'diuretics' can be helpful, too, since cellulite can be made worse by water retention. So along with drinking plenty of water throughout the day, also try dandelion tea and fennel tea, and include cucumbers, celery and asparagus in your diet.

* Nuts contain good fats and are packed with fibre, which is essential for good digestion so that your body can remove all those toxins.

Foods to avoid

* Processed fatty foods, including sausages, cheese, cakes and biscuits, often contain high levels of saturated fats that show up just where we don't want them to, around our bums, love handles and hips.

* Try to keep your intake of coffee and any other caffeine-containing drinks down to one or two a day if possible. Caffeine may inhibit circulation and so reduce the nutrients that reach your skin.

* Cut down on sugar where you can as it may slow the production of collagen in the skin and therefore reduce elasticity, making the appearance of cellulite worse.

Body brushing

This takes just a couple of minutes. Your skin should be dry, so a good time to try this is just before you jump in the shower in the morning. It's a fabulous way to wake up and get your circulation going, which in turn helps your body to eliminate toxins.

✳ Use either a natural bristled brush or loofah, ideally with a nice long handle.

✳ Start with the soles of your feet and then gently brush your legs in an upward motion; think of always brushing towards the heart.

✳ After you brush your legs, brush from the hands along your arms to the shoulders.

✳ Brush upwards on each buttock and then your lower back.

✳ Brush very gently on your stomach, towards the centre.

✳ Finally, brush from the back of your neck around to the front. Don't brush your breasts but you can brush very gently on your chest towards the heart.

So with my bum-busting exercises, body brushing and a clean, fresh diet, you'll soon see those dimples disappearing.

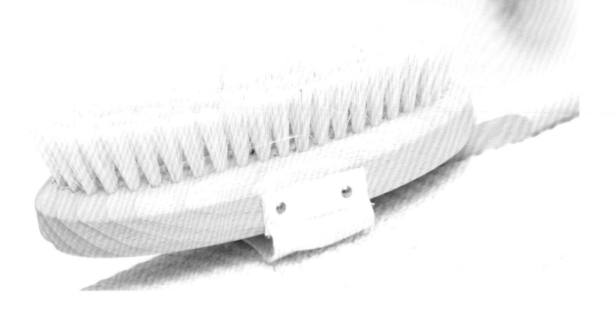

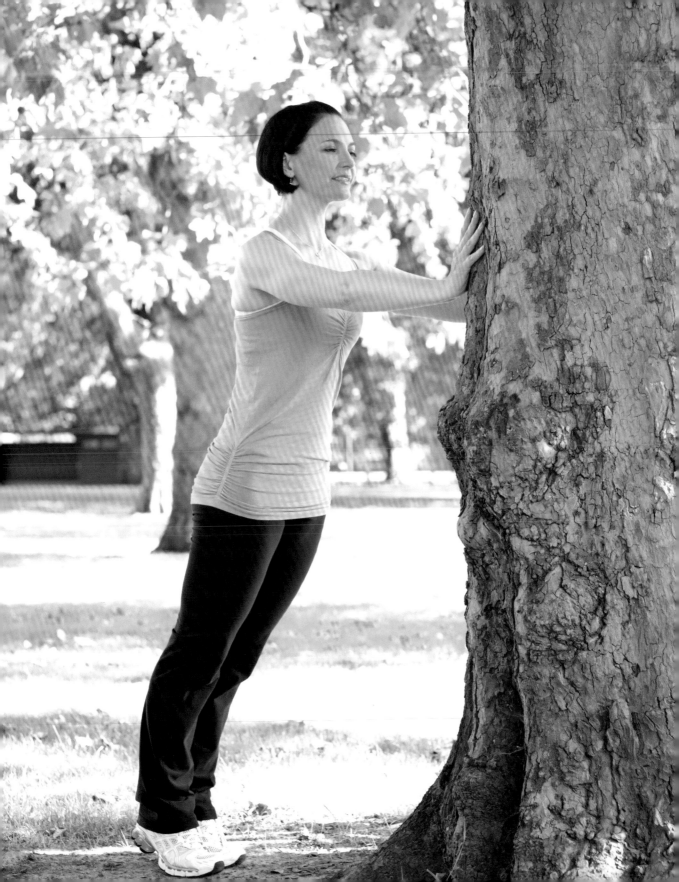

Firing up your motivation

Here one day and somehow gone the next. We all wish we had more willpower and self-control. The thing is that we tend to ask too much of our willpower, which has its limitations, and then feel terrible about ourselves when we don't bother to go to the gym or quickly scoff that second dough-nut. As a Pilates teacher, it's my job to know every motivational trick in the book to feed your willpower, so here are a few of my favourites.

* Focus on the little things, such as your posture (see page 48). Just by sitting, standing and walking straight and tall will boost your positive attitude and so you'll be more likely to grab that band and work on your arms while you wait for the kettle to boil.

* Get into a few healthy habits, such as always walking up escalators rather than just standing there, or having a nice full body stretch (page 57) first thing in the morning, followed by just a few minutes of toning exercises (page 132). These small changes are the best practice you can get for strengthening your willpower.

* If you are feeling a bit stuck, just grab your trainers and do something. It doesn't matter whether it's a squat or getting outside for a quick brisk walk. Starting is the hard part, so don't think about it too much – just get up and do it.

* Set daily goals. Write them down at the beginning of the day and then write down what you have achieved at the end of the day. Focus on what you do manage, not on what you don't. Something is always better than nothing!

* Ask friends and family to help you keep motivated with support and ideas. Encouragement is like a magic tonic for willpower.

* Create some positive affirmations for yourself. I tell myself that I feel great at six o'clock in the morning as I prepare for my first class! Effective affirmations include 'I am energised', 'I am taking care of my body and mind', and 'I am reaching my goals and feeling fabulous'.

Make a commitment here and now. Your health and fitness is important not only for you but for everyone around you. Being healthy lifts your mood, gives you bags more energy and makes you feel more confident. Remember all the benefits and take that first step … or lunge!

'Margot not only makes your whole body work and flex in ways you didn't know were possible but she makes it enjoyable too…' Lucy

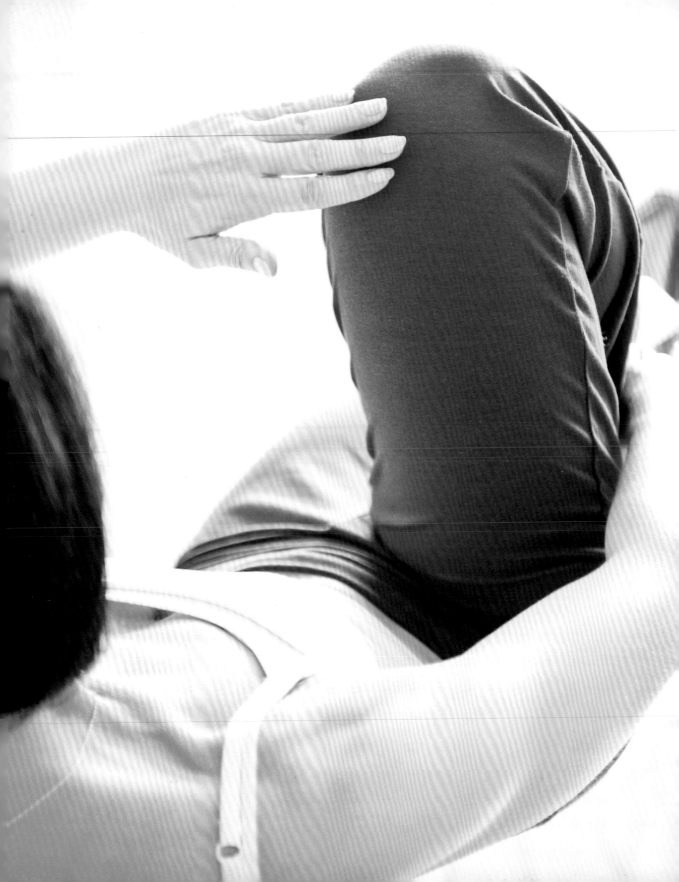

Work your body

The basics

I'm going to take you through an effective exercise programme to strengthen and tone your bottom, your thighs, arms, back and abs. I'll be combining traditional Pilates exercises with other exercises to give you, ultimately, much better definition throughout your body.

For total fitness, combine these routines with other fitness activities to increase your heart rate, for example aerobics, speed walking, skipping, short runs with the baby buggy or cycling, and incorporate as many Cardio on the go activities as you can fit into your day – for example try taking the stairs instead of the lift, abdominal exercises during TV intermissions, or even a few triceps dips on the stairs. This will help you sculpt your way to a better body. But remember that exercise alone won't do it all – you need a healthy diet, too!

Core fitness

Your core muscles, the network of muscles that surround your abdomen, not only help to keep your stomach flat and your waist slim, but are the foundation of good posture, helping you to walk tall and prevent back pain. The stronger your core, the more in control you are of your body, which means that you're able to work the rest of your muscles more effectively.

When you think of your core, see it in imaginary 3D.

The muscles at the front of your stomach are just one piece of the puzzle. Your oblique muscles wrap around your sides and your transversus abdominus gives you strength from inside your body.

Throughout the routines in this book I encourage and remind you to 'draw in your abdominal connection' at your core. I show you how to do this, firstly by learning how to develop and use the breath, and secondly, by forming the navel-to-spine connection while breathing. These are both important when we perform the exercises throughout the book.

'Pilates develops the body uniformly, corrects wrong posture, restores physical vitality, invigorates the mind and elevates the spirit.'
Joseph Pilates

Lifting the head

To complete many of the exercises you will have to lift your head off the mat. It's important to position your head correctly, because if you don't, you will quickly start to experience discomfort in the neck muscles. You don't want to crush your chin to your chest but you do want to lift your head high enough so that you can see your navel. Imagine you are holding a ripe peach gently under your chin, so that it stays in position but doesn't bruise. If your gaze wanders off towards the ceiling, you are probably dropping your neck slightly and straining your neck muscles, so bring your head up a touch and re-focus on your navel.

This position should allow you to complete an exercise without having to release your head halfway through a set of repetitions, or experience any discomfort. However, if you do feel you are straining your neck muscles while doing an exercise, lower your head back down to the mat and move it from one side to the other to relieve the neck. You can then slowly raise it again and continue with the exercise. Other options are not to lift your head at all, or to bring it up on every second repetition. The choice is yours, but if you can, try lifting your head occasionally because this will help to strengthen the neck muscles.

If you do feel discomfort after exercising, try the neck-release exercises on page 180 to help relieve it.

Incorrect neck position

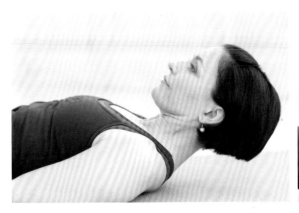

Correct neck position

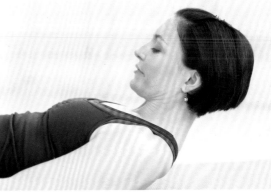

Placement – neutral spine and imprinting

When explaining Pilates exercises throughout this book, I refer to either a neutral or an imprinted spine position.

Finding neutral spine

1. Lie down on your mat and bend your knees to roughly 90 degrees. Feet should be placed flat on the mat, hip-width apart, heels aligned with hips. Place your arms at your sides with your palms resting on the mat. (Arms are raised in the photographs to show the changes in back position.) Lengthen the back of the neck by focusing straight above you, and slightly tuck in the chin. Gently tilt your pelvis back until your lower back touches, or imprints to, the mat. Now try tilting the pelvis forward until your lower back is slightly arched.

2. Gently rock the pelvis back and forward, gradually decreasing the action until you are lying comfortably between these two extremes – your hip bones and pubic bone should be level (imagine you're trying to balance a glass of water on your tummy) and you should have a small natural arch in your lower back. This is your neutral spine position.

3. Now, with your spine still in neutral, try raising your legs one at a time to table-top position, knees bent at 90 degrees. When working in this position you need to maintain a strong navel-to-spine connection in your abdominals to prevent discomfort in your lower back.

Imprinting your spine

1. To imprint your spine from the neutral spine position, all you have to do is slightly tilt the pelvis back, allowing the lower back to touch the mat. This is a very small movement. You are not trying to jam your back into the mat, only imprint it a little. Try this at first with your feet on the mat.

2. Then, with your spine still imprinted, raise your legs one at a time to table-top position, knees bent at 90 degrees. The navel-to-spine connection is easier to maintain in this position as your lower back is slightly supported by the floor.

NOTE

– Maintaining a neutral spine can be quite difficult, especially when you are trying to master the Pilates breathing technique and the navel-to-spine connection while exercising, occasionally causing some lower back discomfort. So for some exercises (mainly when your feet are off the mat) I'll be suggesting that you imprint your spine on the mat, which will provide some additional support for the lower back muscles.

– When you can maintain your neutral spine position with both feet off the mat, you can always challenge yourself by completing a few of each exercise in this position. However, if you feel any discomfort in the lower back muscles, drop back to an imprinted spine position to complete the set. You can always try a few more in neutral spine tomorrow.
– Arms are raised in the photographs to show the changes in back positions.

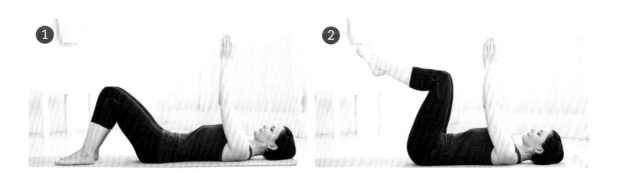

Breathing and forming the navel-to-spine connection

One of the key elements of Pilates is how you use the breath while exercising. Essentially, during most of the exercises, you have to exhale on the effort and draw in your navel-to-spine connection.

The 'navel-to-spine connection' is a phrase I use very early on in my classes because it is the number one thing you have to remember while doing Pilates exercises, and it's also very handy when doing everyday activities too e.g. lifting the baby. During Pilates, the aim is to remain constantly aware of the connection between the pelvic floor muscles, stomach muscles and the breath; this is how we make controlled movements without causing stress to the back. It also means that you flatten your stomach as you exercise and strengthen the abdominals. If you don't pull in your tummy as you exercise, you end up with a taut but slightly protruding stomach.

The best way to understand your navel-to-spine connection is to practise forming the connection while breathing.

1. Standing in front of a mirror, begin by placing your palms on the sides and top of your lower ribcage with your middle fingers slightly touching. Now inhale and exhale naturally, observing any movements of the torso.

2. On your next inhale, breathe deeply into the back of your ribs and observe the movement of the ribs as they flare up and outwards, the middle fingers slightly separating. **This is known as lateral breathing.**

3. As you exhale, contract your lower ribcage inwards. Imagine creating a funnel shape as you feel the ribs move down towards the stomach. At the base of the funnel, zip up the pelvic floor (imagine you are stopping yourself from weeing) and draw your navel in towards your spine, so forming the navel-to-spine connection.

4. Try this a few times, and then have a go at drawing your navel towards your spine so it's 30% of the way in when you finish breathing out – this isn't very much.

Once you have the hang of it, **practise holding on to that 30% connection while flaring and funnelling the ribs as you breathe in and out**, gradually building the navel-to-spine connection from 30% to 40% to 50% and finally to 60%.

NOTE
– *The spine doesn't move when you draw the navel in and you should still be able to breathe, so don't pull in too much!*
– *To prepare for a workout, I recommend you do 5 lateral breaths as you build your navel-to-spine connection to 60%.*

Exhale on the effort and draw in your navel-to-spine connection.

The more you use the abdominal muscles, the less work the lower back muscles have to do and the stronger your core muscles will become.

During the exercises, you'll often be drawing the navel in towards the spine 60%, but for the Plank and Press-ups you'll be drawing in 100%, as far as you can go. So before you begin, it's best to practise drawing in the navel-to-spine connection 30%, 60% and 100% while standing, sitting and lying down, as these will be referred to throughout the workouts. It's important that you master drawing in and holding on to the connection while breathing and performing the exercises. This not only works the abdominal muscles but also stabilises and protects the lower back muscles.

NOTE
– 'Draw in your connection' or 'connect' means the 60% navel-to-spine connection. When I need you to draw your navel to your spine 100%, I will let you know.
– If you are new to Pilates and lateral breathing, you may over-breathe and feel dizzy or light-headed. If this occurs, stop, sit down and breathe normally. As you get used to the deeper breathing technique this should happen less often.

Starting position

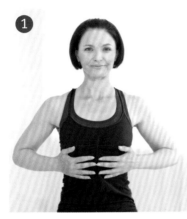

Flaring up and outwards

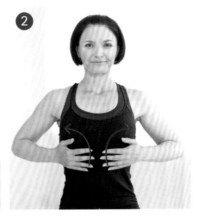

Funelling down and inwards

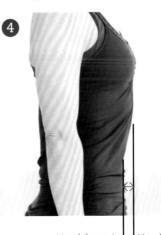

Drawing the navel towards the spine

Navel drawn in | Navel out

It's important that you master drawing in and holding on to the connection while breathing and performing the exercises.

Basic sit-up

Now we are going to try maintaining that 60% navel-to-spine connection while doing a couple of exercises.

1. Begin in a neutral spine position, hands interlaced behind your head. Inhale to prepare and as you exhale, zip up the pelvic floor and draw the navel towards the spine 60%. Inhale and hold on to that connection.

2. Exhale and lift your upper body approximately 4 inches from the mat. Inhale as you lower back down to the mat. Exhale as you lift again. Have a go…

NOTE
– Remember to lift only approximately 4 inches. Any higher and your lower back will press into the mat and you will lose your neutral spine position.

'Both of us feel the positive difference that the sessions have made to our everyday lives. Even walking down the street you hear the mantra 30% or 60%! Our core strength and posture have improved greatly, even after just a few sessions.'
Melissa and Dave

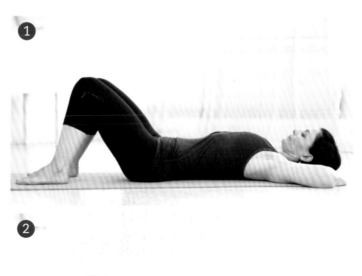

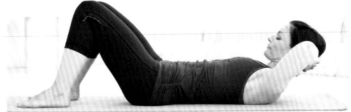

Squat

1. Stand with your feet hip-width apart.

2. Now imagine yourself in the process of sitting down in a chair. Take your weight backwards and into your heels, keeping your knees tracking forward between your big toe and middle toe, with your shoulders down and relaxed, and your arms raised in front of you to just below shoulder height. Breathe in as you lower down. Exhale, zip up your pelvic floor and draw your navel to your spine 60% while pushing back up through the heels to standing, squeezing your thighs and your bottom and making sure your knees don't drift forward beyond your toes.

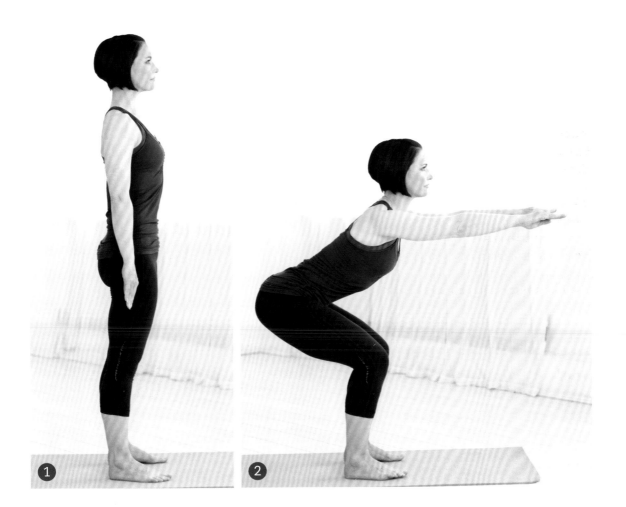

Posture

Before we do anything else I'm going to ask you to have a think about your posture. One of the key areas of Pilates is learning how to lengthen your body and stand correctly, so before we begin our workout I'd like you to consider how you carry yourself in everyday life.

Walk around and notice if, typically, you walk with your head down so that you are looking at the ground in front of you with your shoulders rolling forwards; or do you walk with your shoulders pinned so far back that the area between the shoulder blades aches? Now, stand naturally in front of a mirror and notice what your body is doing. Do you tend to lean over to one side, or perhaps you tend to lock your knees? Stand for a few minutes and your usual habits should become clear.

Now relax and let's reset your posture. Imagine you are standing in a queue and your body is completely relaxed. Set your feet about hip-width apart, and slightly turned out. Soften your knees so that

they are not locked but have just a slight amount of give in them. Centre your weight evenly between your heels and your toes so that you are leaning neither backwards nor forwards but are nicely grounded. Now all that is left for you to do is lift your head and stand up straight. There is no pinching the shoulders back or pushing your chest out. Instead, imagine someone is pulling you up by a thread from the top of your head. Your eye line is level so that your chin is not tilting upwards and your shoulders are resting evenly, neither tensed upwards nor rolling forwards. How does this feel?

Relax again and place the palm of your hand on your stomach. This time as you stand up straight, you should feel your abdominal muscles lifting slightly. You should also notice that your hip bones and pubic bone are aligned, your tailbone is slightly tucked under and there is a natural curve in the base of your spine. You are not trying to flatten your back.

Have another go at this. Remember, you are only lifting your head, your shoulders and back muscles are still relaxed. Learn to recognise this posture and your natural curves in front of a mirror and see how different your body looks.

Simply by standing your height and naturally lifting your abdominal muscles (think 30% navel-to-spine connection) while doing everyday activities, such as walking, will not only help improve your posture, abdominal strength and stability but it will also help relieve some of the pressure on your back muscles as they won't have to work so hard to support you. And furthermore, you'll look great!

There are many other aspects to resetting your posture, but for now, just think of standing your full height while walking as your introduction.

Incorrect position   *Correct position*

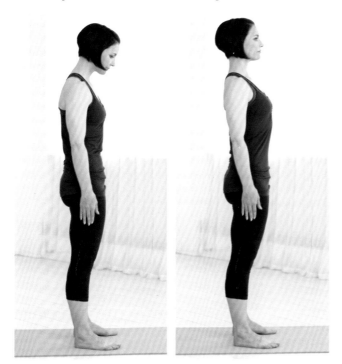

Why not also try resetting your posture while sitting down at your desk and see how this feels.

Incorrect position   *Correct position*

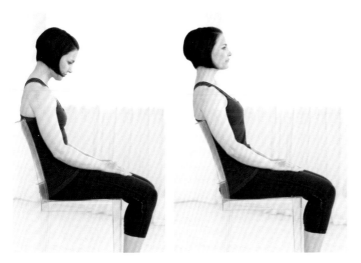

'It's hilarious. Since Margot taught me how to do my pelvic floor exercises, walk my height and form my navel-to-spine connection, I'm doing it in the supermarket, waiting in line at the post office and every time I go for a walk. The little things really do add up and I feel great. Pilates makes you so aware of your body in your daily activities that I now never stand on the escalators, I always walk up them and my legs definitely thank me for it. I feel I have so much more control and poise; and I feel strong but not in a muscular way, just really nicely toned, with far fewer aches and pains and a new-found confidence in my body.' Clare

Pelvic floor

So where exactly is your pelvic floor and what does it do? The pelvic floor in both men and women is a strong muscular sling that connects the pubic bone at the front of the body to the tailbone and sitting bones at the back. Imagine your pelvis is the shape of a mixing bowl with your pelvic floor muscles being layered across this, supporting everything above almost like a hammock. A strong pelvic floor gives you internal core strength while weakness in the pelvic floor muscles can result in a small leakage of urine when you cough, laugh or sneeze, or when you do more vigorous activities, such as Star Jumps and Skipping.

Think of the pelvic floor muscles in two parts, one at the front and one at the back. Therefore you have to exercise both parts. To draw up your pelvic floor muscles at the front, imagine you are stopping the flow of urine (use your imagination – don't do this in practice!). Then try the following exercises.

1. Draw up the pelvic floor muscles and then release them.

REPEAT 10 TIMES.

2. Now draw up the pelvic floor muscles and hold at the top for 5 seconds before releasing them.

REPEAT 5 TIMES.

3. Finally, try drawing up the pelvic floor muscles in stages. Imagine you are in a lift and you are travelling up one floor at a time – try to lift the muscles while travelling at least 4 floors. Once you've reached the top floor, start to drop the muscles one floor at a time until you reach the ground floor and release.

REPEAT 5 TIMES.

Now repeat the exercises at the back. So draw up the anal sphincter (this time imagine you are trying to prevent yourself from breaking wind!) and complete the exercises in just the same way as you did at the front.

If you are planning on doing Star Jumps and Skipping during your fitness and cardio on the go activities, these muscles need to be in tip-top shape. So if you feel they need a little bit of work, practise these exercises every day. They can be done standing, sitting or lying down – any time, any place, anywhere!

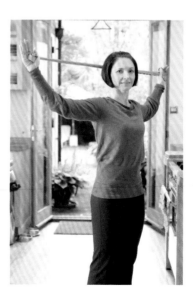

Quick glossary

Adductors: inner thigh muscles.

Biceps: muscles at the front of your upper arms, used for lifting.

Core: the collection of muscles that wrap around your stomach.

Count: the time it takes you to complete a breath, that is one inhalation and one exhalation.

Drawing in your connection: the most important thing to remember as you do the exercises. Draw your navel to your spine either 60% or occasionally 100%, keeping your stomach flat and your core strong.

Glutes (glutei): muscles in your bottom.

Hamstrings: muscles at the back of your legs, running from your knees up to your bottom.

Imprint: a mat position. You tilt your hips just slightly so that your back imprints on the mat. We do most of the exercises in this position to begin with because it is slightly easier than being in the neutral spine position, and protects your lower back while you are gradually strengthening your abdominal muscles.

Navel: your belly button.

Neutral placement: a mat position. When you are lying on the mat with your spine in its neutral position, there will be a slight arch between your spine and the floor.

Obliques: side abdominal muscles, often forgotten, that help to give great definition to your waist.

Pulse: a small repetitive contraction of a muscle at the end of an exercise as you try to fatigue the muscle.

Quads: your front thigh muscles.

Triceps: your underarm muscles, bingo wing territory!

Warm-up

I'm going to start with a gentle warm-up
to improve the mobility and flexibility
of the spine and joints followed by some
lengthening and stretching of the body.
You'll need a mat or a towel, because
there's a fair bit of floor work in the
workouts, and some drinking water. It's
important to keep your fluid levels up and
have a drink whenever you need one. So
when you're ready, let's get started.

Begin by lying down on the mat in a neutral
spine position, with your knees bent. Now
breathe in, flaring the ribs, then funnel them
down gradually building your navel-to-spine
connection to 60% with each lateral breath.
This will form your connection for the rest
of the session. Let's do this 5 more times.

We're now going to start mobilising
the spine.

Pelvic Peeling

1. Begin in a neutral spine position (see page 42), arms at your sides with palms facing upwards to open your shoulders.

2. Inhale to prepare. Exhale, draw in your connection, tilt the pelvis and gently press the lower back into the mat.

3. Then peel one vertebra at a time off the mat up to the mid back, creating a straight line with your body and lengthening through the spine. At the top, breathe in.

4. Exhale as you gradually lower one vertebra at a time to the mat, still maintaining your navel-to-spine connection. Imagine your spine moving like the links of a chain, one link at a time, back to neutral spine position at the bottom.

REPEAT 10 TIMES.

NOTE
— The duration of the exercise from bottom to top should roughly be the length of the exhale. However, if you do run out of air, pause, inhale and then continue to exhale until you reach the top.

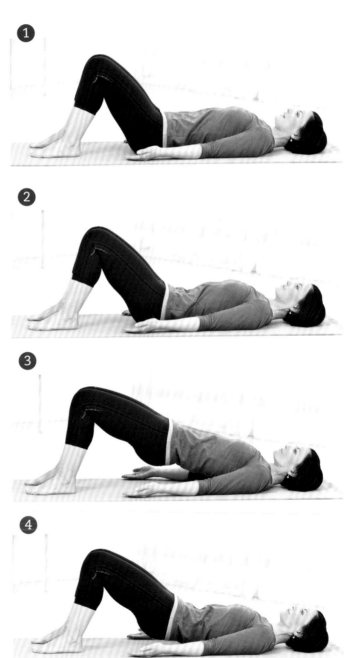

Hip Rolls

1. Begin in a neutral spine position, arms extended out to the sides just below shoulder level with palms facing up. Draw your knees and feet together and lift the heels 1 inch off the mat.

2. Inhale to prepare. Exhale, form your connection and lower your knees to one side, keeping your feet together and both shoulders on the mat, while gently turning your head in the opposite direction. You should feel a nice stretch down the side of the body and in your lower back.

3. Inhale. Exhale, and maintain that navel-to-spine connection as you use your oblique (side) muscles to bring your knees and head back to the centre at the same time. Then repeat on the other side.

REPEAT 5 TIMES ON EACH SIDE.

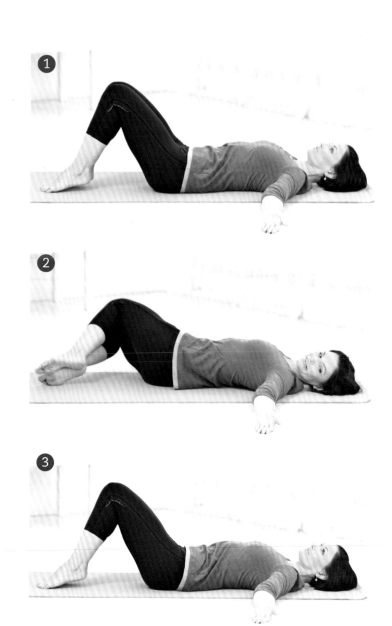

Hip Flexor Stretch

1. Lie on your back in a neutral spine position, legs lengthened along the mat, feet together, arms at your sides.

2. Breathe in and as you breathe out, connect and draw one knee up and into the chest, clasping the knee with both hands.

3. Breathe in again and as you exhale pull the knee in closer. You will feel a slight pinch at the hip. On the next inhale, slightly release the knee and as you exhale draw it in again. Remember, your abdominals are still connected!

4. Repeat 3 times, holding each stretch for the duration of the exhale, and then on the last one rotate the ankle a few times each way to mobilise the ankle joint.

REPEAT ON THE OTHER SIDE.

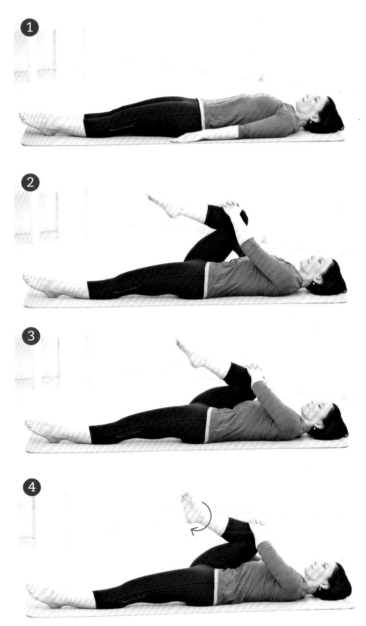

Double Knee Stretch

1. Lie on your back in a neutral spine position, feet together legs lengthened along the mat, with your arms at your sides. Inhale to prepare.

2. Exhale, connect and draw up both legs, one at a time, into the body. Imprint your lower back on the mat, then wrap both arms around your knees. Breathe in and as you exhale, pull your knees in closer to stretch the lower back. Inhale to release the stretch and exhale to deepen it. Repeat 3 times, holding each stretch for a few seconds.

3. On the last repetition, slightly open your knees. Place the palms of your hands on top of them and draw a few circles each way, mobilising the hip joints.

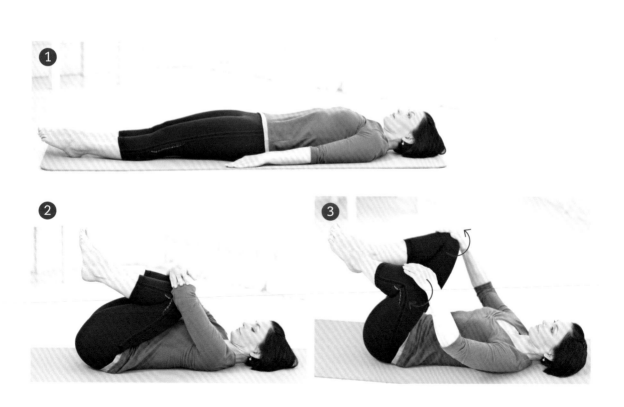

Long Body Stretch

1. Lie on your back, legs lengthened along the mat, arms stretched above your head and shoulders relaxed.

2. Breathe in, and as you exhale stretch your whole body, extending the tips of your fingers and toes, then relax. Inhale again and stretch just the right side of the body as you exhale – remember to stretch the fingers and toes and hold each stretch for the duration of the breath. Repeat on the left side.

3. Finally, stretch the whole body again, but this time slightly arch your ribcage to stretch the front of your abdominals.

NOTE
– This is a lovely full body stretch. Try it the moment you wake up in the morning!

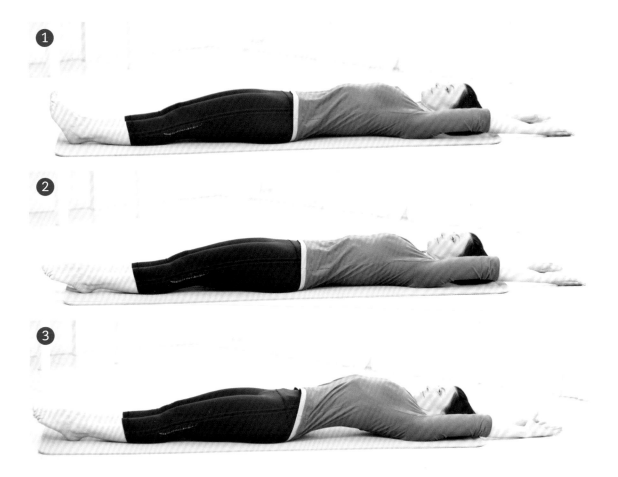

Target Zone: 10 Minute Abdominal Workout

In this workout we're going to focus on sculpting and toning the mid-section of the body by working on the abdominal muscles, often referred to as your core muscles. You'll be flexing, extending and rotating through the spine to improve your core strength.

Start with 8 repetitions of each exercise, building to 12 and, finally, to 16 as you challenge yourself and progress over the weeks.

Basic Starting Position

Lie on your back in a neutral spine position with your knees bent, and let's begin some lateral breathing to build your navel-to-spine connection to 60% (see page 44 if you're unsure).

1. I suggest starting off most of the exercises in the imprinted spine position. Once you're able to perform an exercise easily, try it in a neutral spine position to challenge your abdominals a little more. Drop back into an imprinted spine position if you experience any discomfort in the lower back.

If you feel discomfort in the neck muscles during any of these exercises, lower your head to the mat and gently roll it from side to side to release the tension. Then try raising it again.

2. After you complete each exercise, draw your knees to your chest in a Double Knee Stretch for a few seconds before moving on to the next exercise.

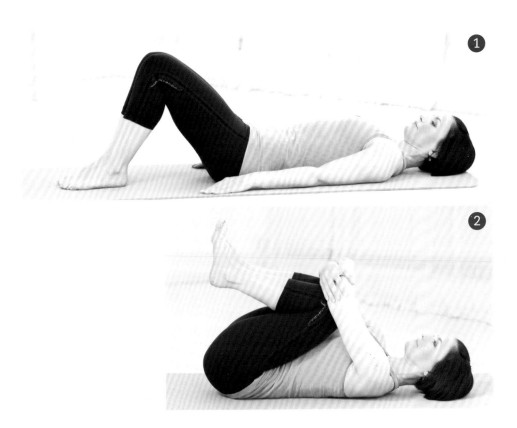

Heel Drops

1. Begin with an imprinted spine, knees in table-top position. Place your arms by your sides, palms facing upwards to open the shoulders.

2. Inhale to prepare. Exhale and connect as you flex from the hip and move one heel slowly towards the mat, maintaining a 90 degree angle at the back of the knee. Don't straighten the leg.

3. Breathe in and as you exhale slowly draw the heel back to table-top position.

REPEAT, SLOWLY, 8 TIMES ON EACH SIDE.

NOTE
– When transitioning from one side to the other, try to maintain the stability of the pelvis by minimising any movements.
– If you feel your lower back is coming off the mat, or you're losing your navel-to-spine connection, you are dropping your heel too far. Start by lowering it just a few inches and gradually increase this as you find the exercise getting easier.

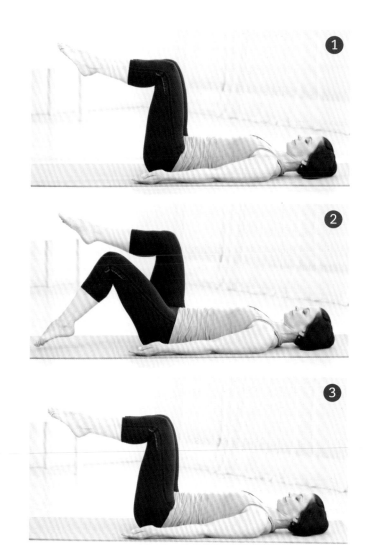

Leg Extensions

1. Begin with an imprinted spine, knees in table-top position. Inhale, cradle your head in your hands and lift the head. Elbows are wide.

2. Exhale, connect and gently extend one leg to a 45 degree angle with the mat.

3. Breathe in and as you exhale, slowly bring the leg back to the start position. Repeat with the other leg.

REPEAT, SLOWLY, 8 TIMES ON EACH SIDE, KEEPING EACH LEG EXTENDED FOR 2 SECONDS.

NOTE
– The head should remain cradled in the hands throughout this movement, and the neck muscles should be completely relaxed.
– When transitioning from one side to the other, try to maintain the stability of the pelvis by minimising any movements.
– If you feel your lower back is coming off the mat, or you're losing your navel-to-spine connection, try taking the legs higher as you extend them. Once you can maintain the connection, take them lower again to challenge yourself.

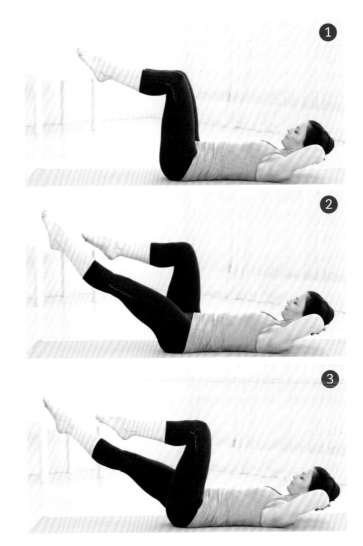

The Hundred

1. Begin with an imprinted spine, knees in table-top position, arms by your sides.

2. Breathe in to prepare and as you exhale, connect and curl your head and shoulders off the mat. Lift your arms about 4 inches, palms facing down.

3. Using short inhales, pump your arms up and down 5 times. Imagine you are splashing them in water. Using short exhales, continue to pump your arms up and down, another 5 times.

Repeating this cycle 10 times, equals 100 arm pumps – hence the name of the exercise.

4. To challenge yourself, extend your legs up to 90 degrees.

5. As you breathe in and pump your arms, lower your legs about 6 inches, keeping the toes pointed.

6. As you exhale, continue to pump your arms, slightly turn out the legs from the hips and flex the feet. Then bring the legs back to the centre, really

working the lower abdominal muscles.

REPEAT THE CYCLE 10 TIMES.

NOTE
– *Try to maintain the stability of the pelvis throughout this exercise. If you feel your lower back is coming off the mat, or you're losing your navel-to-spine connection, try drawing the knees closer to your body.*
– *Be careful not to over-breathe! If you feel light-headed, take a break.*

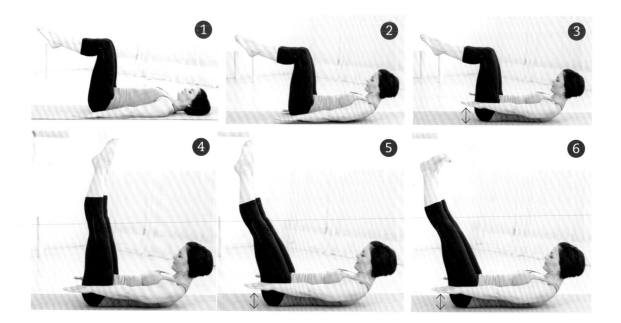

Single Leg Stretch

1. Begin with an imprinted spine, knees in table-top position, arms by your sides.

2. Breathe in to prepare and as you exhale, connect, curl your head and shoulders off the mat and extend your left leg to a 45 degree angle with the mat, drawing your right knee in towards your chest. Tap your right hand to the outside of the ankle on the bent leg and left hand to the top of this knee. Keep your elbows open and high throughout and focus on your navel.

3. Inhale, and as you exhale change legs. Extend your right leg 45 degrees and draw your left knee in towards your chest. Tap your left hand to the outside of the ankle on the bent leg and right hand to the top of this knee. Keep your elbows open and high throughout and focus on your navel.

REPEAT, SLOWLY, 8 TIMES ON EACH LEG.

NOTE
– This is a tricky exercise to master. So if you get the hand positions confused, lower the head back to the mat and continue the exercise until you master the hands and legs. Then lift your head again and focus on the navel. Hopefully, this will prevent any discomfort in the neck.
– Try to maintain the stability of the pelvis. If you feel your lower back is coming off the mat, or you're losing your navel-to-spine-connection, try lifting the legs higher.

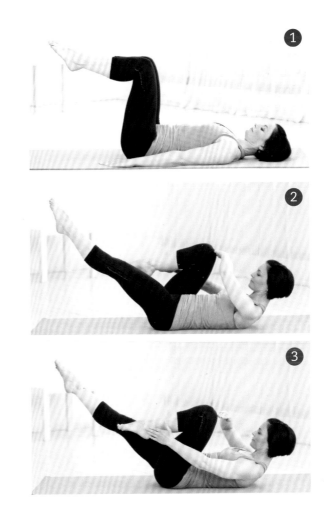

Single Straight Leg Stretch

1. Begin with an imprinted spine, knees in table-top position. Then extend both legs towards the ceiling, toes pointed.

2. Inhale to prepare and as you exhale, connect and curl your head and shoulders up, and split the legs, bringing the right leg towards you. Position your hands behind your right ankle or calf muscle, depending on your flexibility and how far you can reach.

3. Inhale. Exhale, pull your right leg towards you and lower your left leg to 45 degrees. As you draw the right leg in, pulse for 2 quick beats (one, two), exhaling twice as you beat (it's easier if you count aloud). Keep your shoulders down and relaxed and your abs connected. Then switch legs, drawing your left leg in and pulse for 2. Keep alternating between legs.

REPEAT 8 TIMES ON EACH SIDE.

NOTE
– If you are unable to straighten your legs due to very tight hamstrings, come back to this exercise at a later date, once you've stretched those muscles.

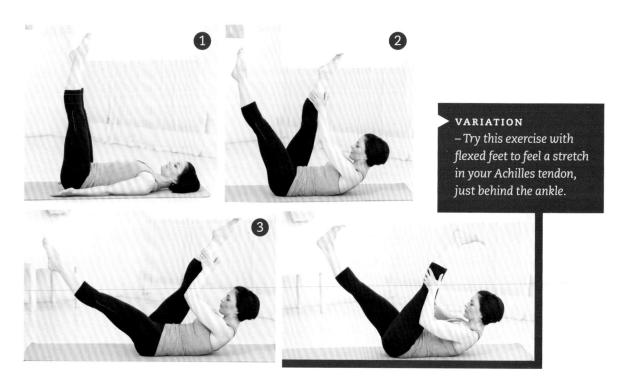

VARIATION
– Try this exercise with flexed feet to feel a stretch in your Achilles tendon, just behind the ankle.

Criss Cross

1. Begin with an imprinted spine, knees in table-top position. Cradle your head in your hands, keep your shoulders relaxed and elbows wide.

2. Breathe in to prepare and as you exhale, connect and rotate your upper body, lifting your right shoulder to meet your left knee, which you draw in towards you, keeping the pelvis still, elbows wide and shoulders down. As you draw in the left knee, lengthen the right leg to 45 degrees. As you inhale, come back to the start position, lowering your upper body completely to the mat before repeating the move on the other side.

REPEAT, SLOWLY, 8 TIMES ON EACH SIDE.

NOTE
– Remember to maintain the navel-to-spine connection throughout, keep your elbows wide, and drop your upper body (including your head) to the mat before you move from one side to the other.

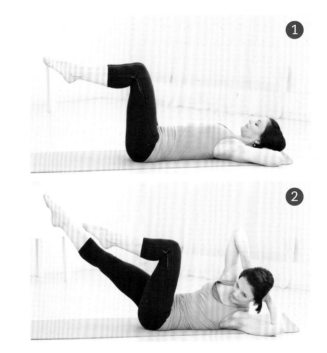

SIMPLIFY
– If you are unable to maintain the stability of the pelvis throughout this exercise, lower your feet to the mat and try lifting the opposite knee to meet the opposite shoulder from here.

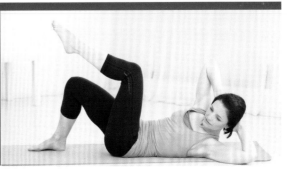

Double Leg Lower and Lift

1. Begin with an imprinted spine, knees in table-top position then extend both legs towards the ceiling, toes pointed. Cradle your head in your hands and lift, keeping elbows wide.

2. Inhale to prepare and as you exhale, connect and slowly lower the legs 6 to 12 inches, keeping your back imprinted on the mat.

3. Breathe in, turn out your legs from the hips and flex your feet.

4. Exhale and draw the legs back to centre, keeping your elbows wide and shoulders open.

REPEAT, SLOWLY, 8 TIMES, KEEPING THE HEAD RAISED THROUGHOUT.

NOTE
– *Try to maintain the stability of the pelvis. If you feel your lower back is coming off the mat, or you're losing your navel-to-spine connection, try lowering the legs just a few inches before turning the legs out, flexing the feet and drawing the legs back up to the centre.*
– *If you are unable to straighten your legs due to tightness in the hamstrings, place a small cushion under your lower back. This will help you to straighten the legs and relieve some of the tension in legs and back.*

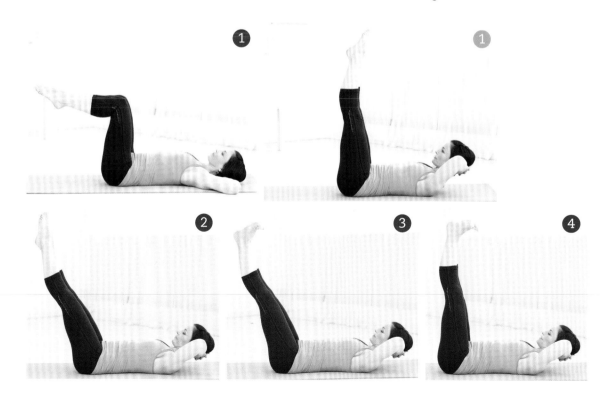

Parallel Abdominals

1. Begin with an imprinted spine, knees in table-top position, arms extended above the chest, palms facing down. Keep your shoulders down and relaxed.

2. Inhale to prepare and as you exhale, connect and slowly press your arms to the sides of your body (imagine you are pushing through treacle) while lifting your head and extending your legs, lowering them 6 to 12 inches away from your body, in one gentle fluid movement.

3. Inhale and slowly reverse the movement, bringing the body back to the start position. Think of the inhale as your rest before your next repetition, so don't rush the descent!

REPEAT, SLOWLY, 8 TIMES.

NOTE
– Try to maintain the stability of the pelvis. If you feel your lower back is coming off the mat or you're losing your navel-to-spine connection, try extending the legs straight up or just keep them at table-top position throughout the exercise.
– If you feel any tension in the neck muscles while the head is raised, lower your head to the mat and gently roll it from side to side to release the tension. Then try bringing it up on every second repetition.

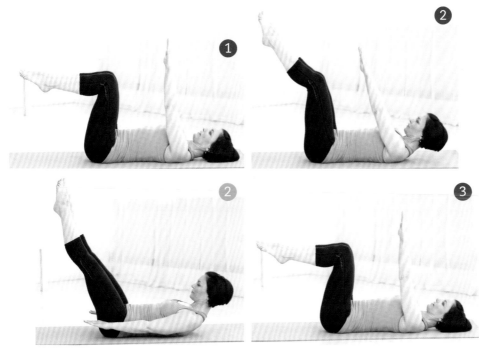

Double Leg Stretch

1. Begin with an imprinted spine, knees in table-top position. Breathe in to prepare and as you exhale, connect, curl your head and shoulders off the mat, tuck in your chin and focus on your navel. Lift your hands to either side of the knees.

2. Breathe in and take your arms back to the sides of the ears and extend your legs away from the body, keeping the toes pointed and the back imprinted to the mat.

3. Breathe out and slowly circle your arms back to the sides of the legs, returning the legs to table-top position.

REPEAT 8 TIMES, KEEPING HEAD AND SHOULDERS STILL AND LIFTED THROUGHOUT.

NOTE
— *Try to maintain the stability of the pelvis. If you feel your lower back is coming off the mat or you're losing your navel-to-spine connection, try extending the legs straight up.*
— *Try not to draw the knees closer to the body as you bring them back to table-top position.*

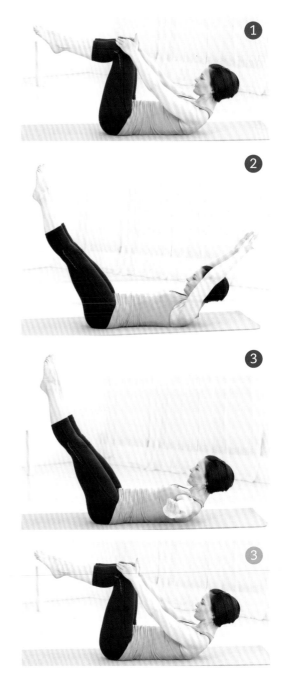

Roll-up with a Twist

1. Begin in a neutral spine position. Breathe in and lift the arms above the chest towards the ceiling, palms facing inwards. Extend your legs one at a time along the mat and flex your feet.

2. Exhale, connect, tuck in your chin and curl the upper body off the mat, one vertebra at a time, keeping your shoulders back and down.

3. Try squeezing the inner thighs together and flexing your feet as you curl up to 90 degrees, using your abdominal strength. Pause at the top and imagine you are being pulled up by a thread through the top of your head – try not to collapse in the upper body.

4. Breathe in and as you exhale, very slowly twist from the waist to one side, keeping the arms extended in front of the chest, palms facing each other throughout. Breathe in and on the exhale return to the centre. Repeat on the other side.

5. Inhale and as you exhale, roll back down in a controlled movement, using your abdominal strength. Keep squeezing the inner thighs and flexing your feet – this will help you to control your descent.

REPEAT 8 TIMES.

NOTE
– As you twist at the top of this movement, don't let your arms wander off. Focus on twisting from your waist and as you twist your arms will move with your torso.
– Remember to maintain the navel-to-spine connection and keep the shoulders back and down throughout this exercise.
– If you find this exercise difficult to begin with, try it with your legs slightly bent.

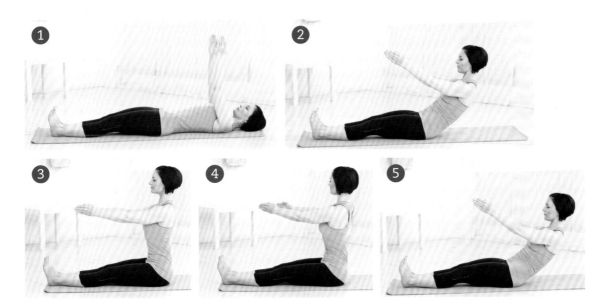

Open Leg Rocker

1. Begin by sitting on the mat with knees bent at 90 degrees and feet separated. Place both hands just behind the knees on the thighs. Shoulders are relaxed.

2. Inhale to prepare and as you exhale, connect and gently round the spine as you tilt the pelvis back and rest on your bottom. Lift the feet about 6 inches off the mat and point your toes.

3. Inhale and roll back on to the upper back, straightening your legs into a v-shape and pointing your toes.

4. Exhale, contract your abdominal muscles and roll forward to the start position, keeping your legs extended. Hold the position for 2 seconds.

REPEAT 8 TIMES. ON THE LAST REPETITION, HOLD AT THE TOP FOR 5 SECONDS.

NOTE
– If you are unable to extend your legs fully, try doing the exercise with your knees bent.
– Remember to maintain the navel-to-spine connection and keep the shoulders back and down throughout this exercise.

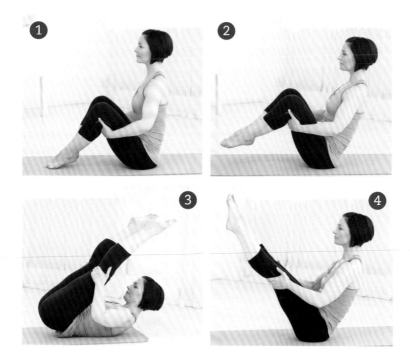

Long Body Stretch

1. Lie on your back, legs lengthened along the mat, arms stretched above your head and shoulders relaxed. Breathe in, and as you exhale stretch your whole body, extending the tips of your fingers and toes, then relax. Inhale again and stretch just the right side of the body as you exhale – remember to stretch the fingers and toes and hold each stretch for the duration of the breath. Repeat on the left side.

2. Finally, stretch the whole body again, but this time slightly arch your ribcage to stretch the front of your abdominals.

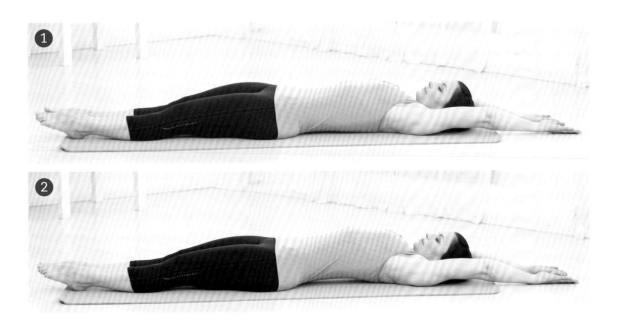

Target Zone:
10 Minute
Back, Arms and
Chest Workout

The main aim of this workout is to tone and strengthen your back muscles, which work together with your abdominal muscles to help sculpt the mid-section. You'll also be working the arms and chest. Throughout this workout, you'll be flexing and extending the spine to improve your back strength. As with the abdominal exercises, start with 8 repetitions, building to 12 and, finally, to 16.

Box Press-up

We'll start with Press-ups, which work the upper body and tone the chest and the triceps. You need to maintain a 100% navel-to-spine connection throughout this exercise, and move the body as a whole, staying in a straight line.

I've included three versions, each more challenging than the last. Try to do 4 of each one, dropping back down to an easier option if you need to. You are aiming to complete 12 Press-ups in total. I recommend that you try a couple of the Full Press-ups, even if at the beginning you can lower yourself only a few inches. You will quickly improve with practice, and these are fantastic exercises for the whole body.

Ok, so when you're ready, come down to an all-fours position.

1. Place your palms directly under your shoulders and then take them slightly wider than shoulder width. Your back is flat, lengthen the neck (imagine your hands as the base of a triangle, your gaze should be focused on the apex of the triangle just ahead of you) and position your knees below the hips.

2. Breathe in to prepare. Exhale and draw in your connection 100%. Inhale as you bend your elbows to drop down towards the mat.

3. Exhale as you push back up through the heel of your hands.

NOTE
– Remember to move your whole body as one, and don't forget that 100% connection.

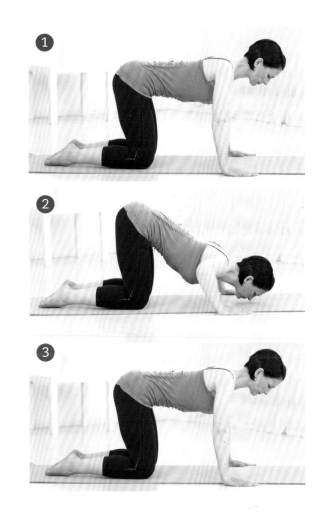

Half Press-up

1. To move into a Half Press-up position, take your knees back one at a time, lift your head and move the body slightly forward in line with the shoulders, lowering your bottom to create a diagonal line from the base of your spine to your head. Your palms are slightly wider than shoulder-width, and your back is flat. Remember to lengthen the neck and draw the navel to the spine 100%.

2. Breathe in as you bend your elbows, keeping your body in a nice straight line, and almost touch the mat.

3. Exhale, and push up through the chest, back of the arms and shoulders to the start position.

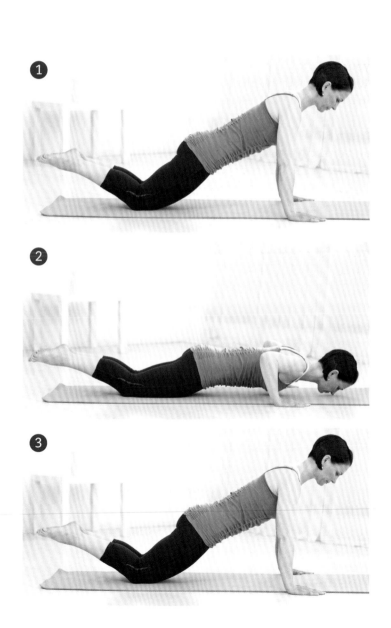

Full Press-up

1. To move into a Full Press-up position, extend one leg back followed by the other, toes tucked under. Lengthen the neck (remember the triangle, page 73) and draw your navel to your spine 100%. Your body should be in a diagonal line.

2. Inhale, bend the elbows and drop down in between the hands keeping your body taut and in a straight line as you descend.

3. Exhale as you push back up, pressing through your palms and making sure to keep that 100% connection.

Now drop your knees, sit back on your heels and prepare for the Shell Stretch.

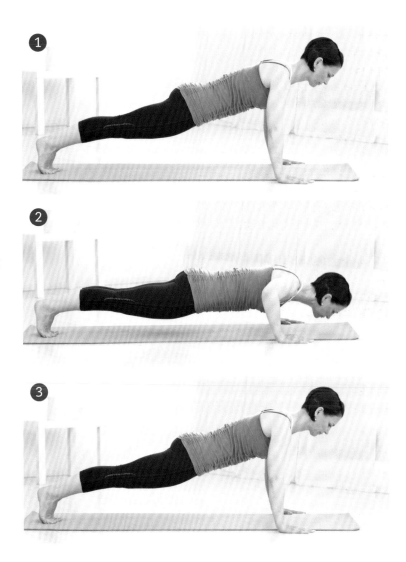

Shell Stretch

1. Begin in an all-fours position and then push back on to your heels with your back rounded and hands in front of you to give your arms, shoulders and back a nice stretch. Breathe in to prepare. Exhale, connect and let your bottom sink down towards your heels. Take 3 deep breaths in and out, and with each exhale drop deeper into the stretch.

2. Do this first with your knees together and then open them slightly to allow the upper body a deeper stretch.

Sit up, and prepare for a Chest and Shoulder Stretch.

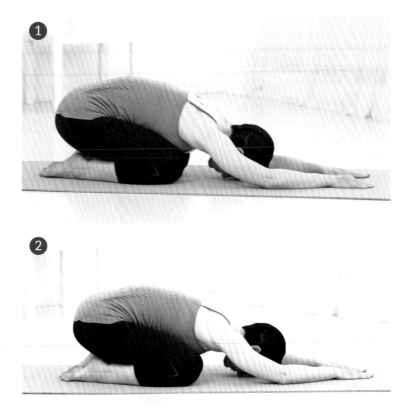

Chest and Shoulder Stretch

1. Sit on your heels, looking straight ahead with your chest high, shoulders relaxed and palms resting on the front of the legs.

2. Breathe in, and as you exhale connect, and extend your arms out to the sides to open and stretch the front of your chest and shoulders.

REPEAT 3 TIMES AND HOLD EACH STRETCH FOR THE DURATION OF THE BREATH.

Now tuck your toes under and roll up to standing and prepare for some arm work.

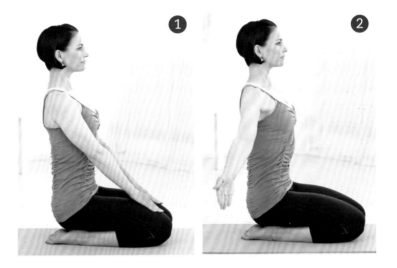

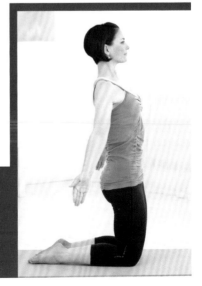

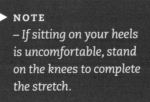

NOTE
– If sitting on your heels is uncomfortable, stand on the knees to complete the stretch.

Lat Pull Downs

1. Wrap the band around your hands for a good grip and to create some tension in it. Begin with your arms above your head, palms facing forward and your feet hip-width apart. Keep your knees soft and have some weight in your heels; don't tip forward.

2. Breathe in, and as you exhale, connect and pull the band out to the sides, lowering it to the front of your chest while bringing the elbows down towards the ribcage. Don't lock your elbows at the bottom of the movement – they should still be slightly bent – and keep your wrists strong.

3. Inhale as you return to the start position.

REPEAT 8 TIMES.

NOTE
– Try not to lose the tension in the band between repetitions.

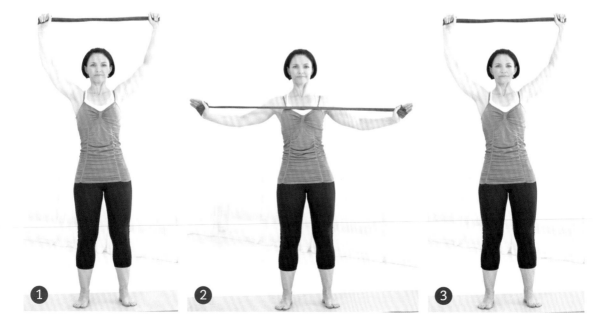

Chest Extensions

1. From the same starting position as Lat Pull Downs, take the band behind your head.

2. Breathe in, and as you exhale, connect and extend your elbows to lower the band down to your bottom. Keep the band close to your back as you go down.

3. Inhale, and on the exhale, bend your elbows again to bring the band back up behind your head to the start position.

REPEAT 8 TIMES.

NOTE
– Try to keep your shoulders and arms moving evenly throughout this exercise, and try not to lose the tension in the band.

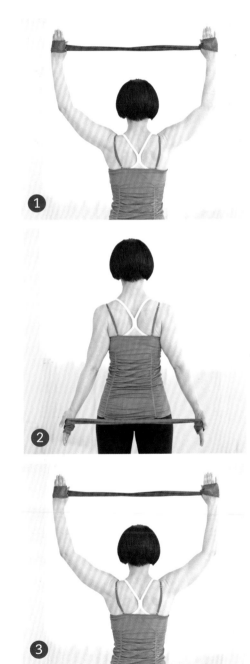

Triceps Extensions

1. Start in the same position as for Lat Pull Downs, but release a little tension in the band. Take your left hand behind your back, placing the back of your hand against your waist. Holding on to the band, and taking care to stand tall, bend your right arm over your head.

2. Breathe in, and as you exhale, connect and straighten your right arm upwards, keeping your upper arm glued to the side of your head.

3. Come back to the start position on the inhale.

REPEAT 8 TIMES ON EACH SIDE, MAINTAINING THE TENSION IN THE BAND.

Now roll down and lie on your tummy and prepare for the Cobra.

NOTE
– To make this exercise harder on your triceps, lower the arm behind your back; and to make it a little easier, simply raise your hand a touch to release tension in the band.

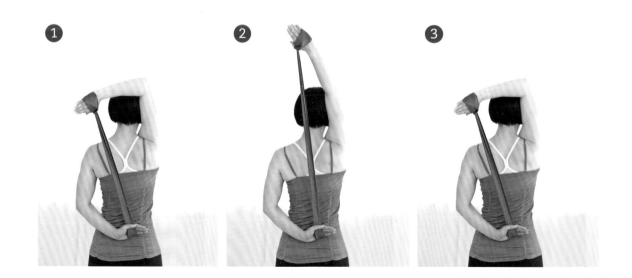

Cobra

1. Lie on your front, neck long, legs hip-width apart and extended along the mat, hands level with your head, palms and elbows on the mat.

2. Breathe in to prepare. Exhale, connect and lift your hands and head off the mat, keeping your chest open for the duration of the exhale. Keep lengthening through the top of your head and looking down towards the mat.

3. Inhale as you gently lower back to the start position.

REPEAT 8 TIMES AND REMEMBER THAT CONNECTION.

NOTE
– *This exercise works the upper portion of your back, so don't be tempted to tighten your bottom or raise your legs.*
– *If you feel discomfort in the lower back, place a small cushion under your tummy and draw in your connection.*

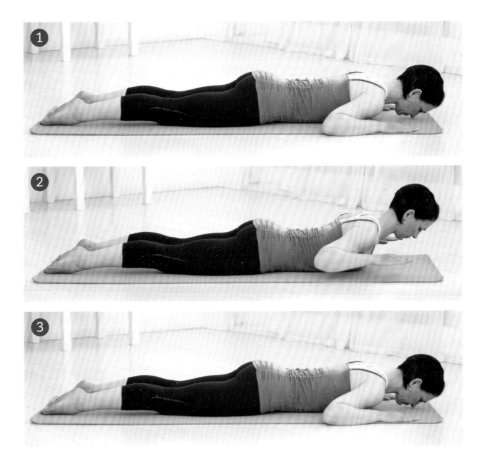

Dart with Arm Beats

1. Still lying on your front, lengthen your neck and extend your arms along your sides, turn your palms up towards the ceiling, legs extended, feet together and toes pointed.

2. Breathe in to prepare. Exhale, connect and lift your head, shoulders, hands and feet off the mat.

3. Inhale and using short exhales, beat your hands together towards the centre of your back for 10 beats. Keep lengthening through the top of your head and looking down towards the mat.

4. Inhale and come back to the start position to relax for a few seconds before repeating.

REPEAT 8 TIMES.

NOTE
– If you feel discomfort in the lower back, place a small cushion under your tummy and draw in your connection.

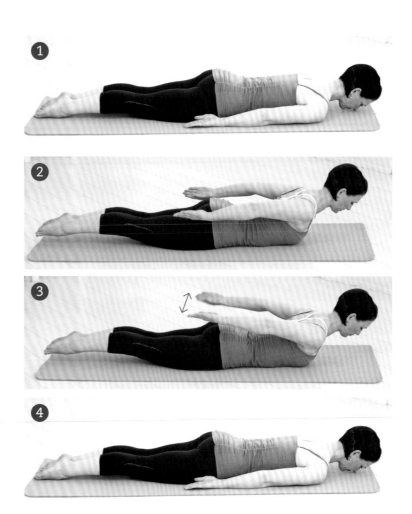

Swimming

1. Still on your front, extend your arms and legs along the mat, palms down, shoulders relaxed and feet hip-width apart.

2. Breathe in to prepare. Exhale, connect and lift your head, and opposite arm and leg a couple of inches off the mat. Use short exhales while alternately raising opposite arms and legs in a swimming motion, resting each arm and leg lightly on the mat before changing to the other side. Remember to keep your tummy drawn in.

3. Once you've mastered the move, try completing the exercise a little faster without resting on the mat as you move from one side to the other. Swim for 16 counts, then come back to the start position for a couple of seconds rest.

REPEAT FOR 3 SETS OF 16 COUNTS.

Now push back on to your knees into the Shell Stretch (page 76) to give your arms, shoulders and back a nice stretch. Do this first with your knees together and then open them slightly and let your bottom sink deeper as you exhale. Now sit up.

NOTE
– Don't lift your arms and legs too high – just a few inches. Your pelvis shouldn't be rocking from side to side.
– If you feel discomfort in the lower back, place a small cushion under your tummy and draw in your connection.

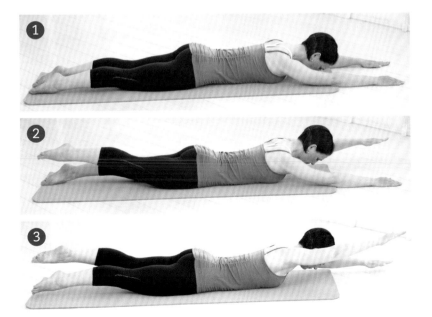

The Kitty Cat

1. Begin on all-fours, your hands slightly wider than your shoulders, your knees directly under your hips and your pelvis in neutral. Your back is flat and your neck long (remember the triangle, page 73).

2. Breathe in to prepare and as you exhale, connect and drop your head forward, arch the upper back and feel your tailbone tucking under.

3. Move your bottom back towards your heels, feeling the stretch through the spine as you move.

4. Inhale as you bend the elbows out to the sides and skim your nose along the mat until your face passes through your hands.

5. Exhale, drop your head, push up and arch the upper back to begin again.

REPEAT 8 TIMES.

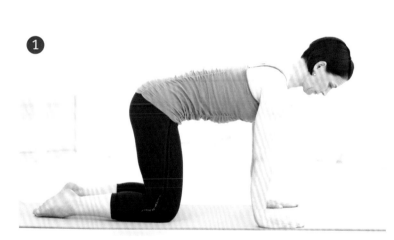

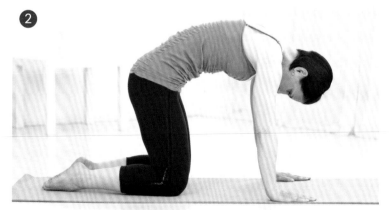

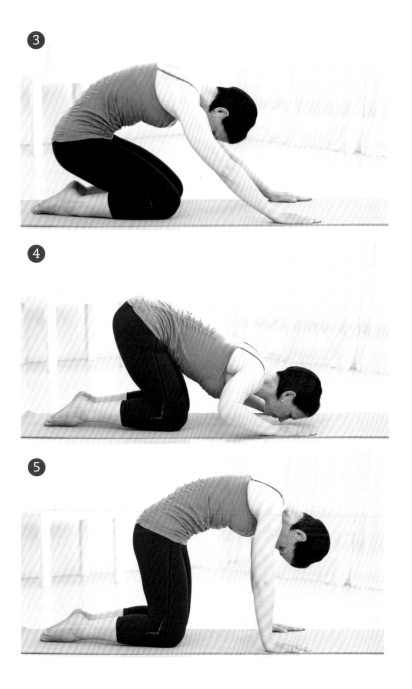

Triceps Dips

1. Sit on the mat, knees bent, feet together. Place your hands to the side of and just behind your bottom, fingers facing forwards.

2. Breathe in as you bend your elbows back and lower your upper body towards the mat.

3. Exhale, connect and push back up to the start position, pressing through the palms of your hands and keeping your body straight, neck lengthened and relaxed.

COMPLETE 2 SETS OF 8 REPETITIONS.

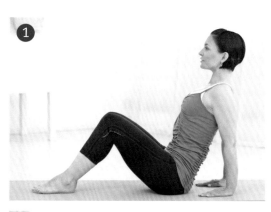

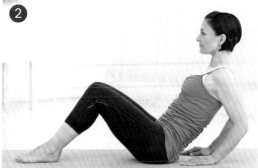

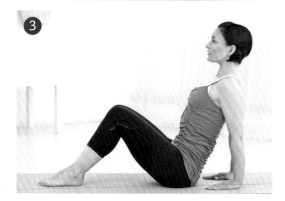

VARIATION
— *To challenge yourself, lift your bottom 2 inches off the mat while performing the dips.*

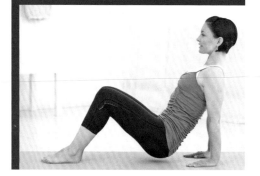

Half Plank

1. Begin on all-fours with your hands directly under your shoulders and neck lengthened (remember the triangle, page 73).

2. Extend one knee back followed by the other and lift your feet off the mat. Drop your bottom to create a straight diagonal line with your body. Draw your connection in 100%. Breathe in for a count of 2, and exhale for a count of 2 as you push away from the mat with the heels of your hands.

HOLD THE POSITION FOR 2 LOTS OF 30 SECONDS.

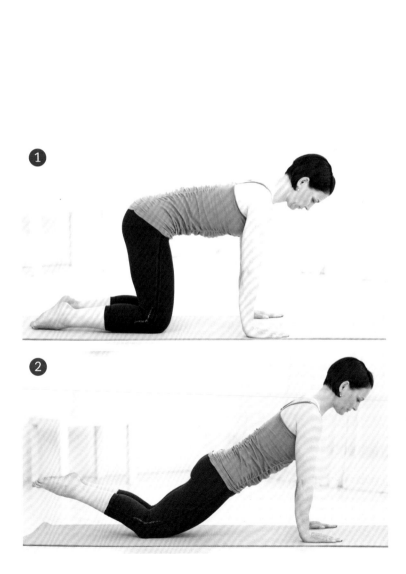

Full Plank

1. From the Half Plank position, tuck your toes under and lift your knees to create a long diagonal line with your whole body.

2. Remember to keep 100% connection and lengthen the neck. Breathe in for a count of 2 and out for a count of 2, pressing away from the mat with the heels of your hands.

HOLD THE POSITION FOR 2 LOTS OF 30 SECONDS.

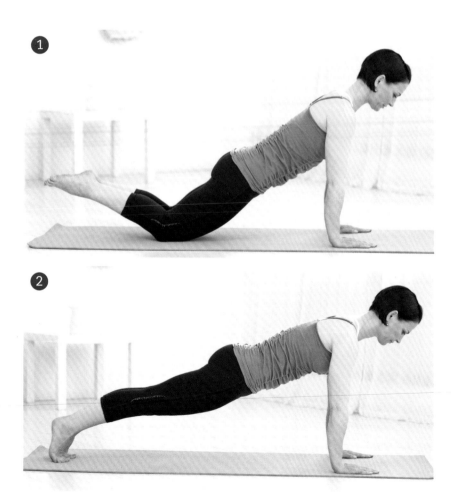

Side Plank

1. Turn on to your side, bending your knees at 90 degrees and resting on your elbow, which should be positioned directly under your shoulder. Extend your other arm down the side of your body. Split your feet so that your top foot is on the mat, just ahead of your bottom foot; this will give you better balance.

2. With legs still bent, breathe in to prepare. Exhale, connect 100% and lift your body up, raising the top arm straight above your shoulder. Hold for 30 seconds. Reverse the movement back to the start position as you breathe in.

REPEAT TWICE ON EACH SIDE.

3. To make this more challenging, try it with straight legs.

4. For the ultimate challenge, try it with straight legs and a straight lower arm.

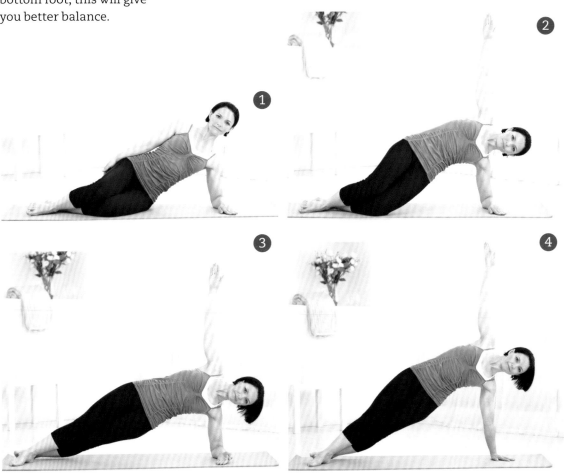

Stretches

As you do these stretching exercises, imagine breathing in to the areas and muscles you are stretching, and as you exhale press a little more, but gently, to increase the stretch.

NOTE
– All the stretches are shown in a kneeling position, but they can also be done standing or in a seated position.

Shoulder Stretch

1. Sit on your heels and stretch your right arm straight across your body, palm open. Place your left hand on your right upper arm. Inhale to prepare, and as you exhale, connect and draw the arm towards you. Feel the stretch in the back of the shoulder. Hold each stretch for a few seconds before release.

REPEAT 3 TIMES ON EACH SIDE.

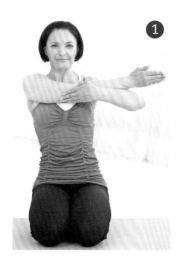

Triceps Stretch

1. Sit on your heels and take your right arm up behind your head, placing the palm of your hand in between your shoulder blades. Take your left arm up and over to grasp the right elbow.

2. Breathe in and then exhale, connect and press down on the elbow to stretch the back of the arm. Hold for a few seconds before release.

REPEAT 3 TIMES ON EACH SIDE.

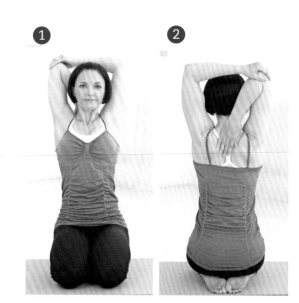

Upper Back Stretch

1. Sit on your heels, take your arms out in front of you and clasp your fingers together.

2. Inhale, and as you exhale, connect and gently push your hands away from the body,

holding the stretch for a few seconds before releasing. You should feel this stretch across the upper back and at the base of the shoulders.

REPEAT 3 TIMES.

3. On the final breath drop your head for a deeper stretch.

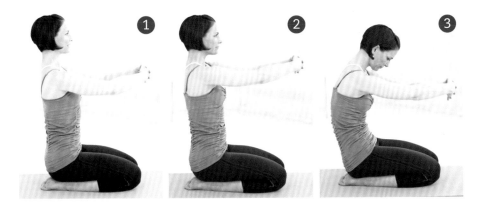

Chest Stretch

1. Sit on your heels and clasp your hands behind your back while keeping your neck and shoulders relaxed and your back straight.

2. Inhale to prepare. Exhale, connect and lift your arms behind you until you feel the stretch across the chest. Hold for a few seconds before releasing.

REPEAT 3 TIMES.

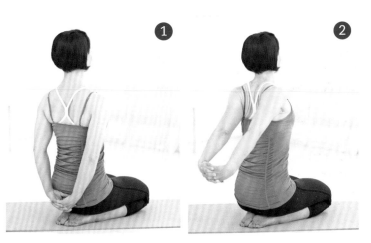

Target Zone: 10 Minute Bottom and Thighs Workout

In this workout we're going to concentrate on toning and strengthening the glutes (glutei muscles in your bottom) and the surrounding area to help lift and improve the shape of your legs and bottom.

Start with 8 repetitions of each exercise, building to 12 and, finally, to 16.

Shoulder Bridge

1. Lie on your back in a neutral spine position with legs comfortably bent, feet hip-width apart and palms facing upwards to open the shoulders.

2. Breathe in and as you exhale, connect and then lift your bottom straight up to create a straight diagonal line with your body, working your glutes and hamstrings. Hold for 2 seconds at the top, then lower down.

REPEAT 8 TIMES, KEEPING YOUR CONNECTION THROUGHOUT.

'I'm pretty fit and eat healthily but I always wanted to improve the tone of my thighs and, to be honest, my bottom. Pilates to the rescue! After just a few sessions I can really feel and now see the difference. I can't wait to wear my bikini this summer.' Victoria

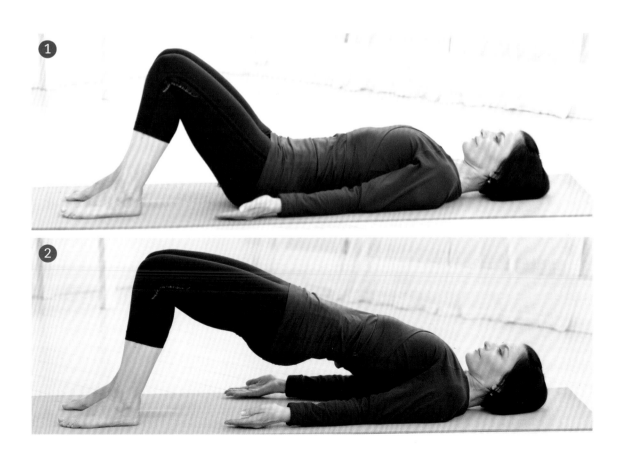

Leg Lifts

1. Lie on your front with your forehead resting on the backs of your hands.

2. Breathe in to prepare. On the exhale, connect and lift one leg up for a count of 2, then slowly lower it for a count of 2 as you breathe in again and prepare for the next lift. Alternate legs and repeat 8 times on each side.

Repeat the exercise, but this time lift and lower on single counts, so it's a bit quicker. Remember to keep your connection drawn in 60%.

3. Finally, lift both legs, squeeze your glutes together, and beat your legs for 3 sets of 12. Beat from the upper inner thighs, keeping the knees straight.

NOTE
– If you feel discomfort in the lower back, place a small cushion under your tummy and check you're still drawing in your connection.

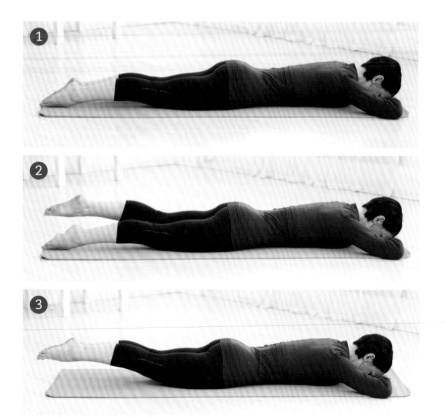

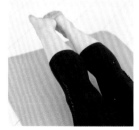

Beat your legs

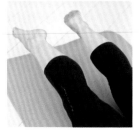

Shell Stretch

1. Push back on to your heels with your back rounded and hands in front of you to give your arms, shoulders and back a nice stretch.

2. Breathe in, and as you exhale, connect and let your bottom sink down towards your heels. Take 3 deep breaths in and out, dropping deeper into the stretch with each exhale.

Do this first with your knees together and then open them slightly to allow the upper body a deeper stretch.

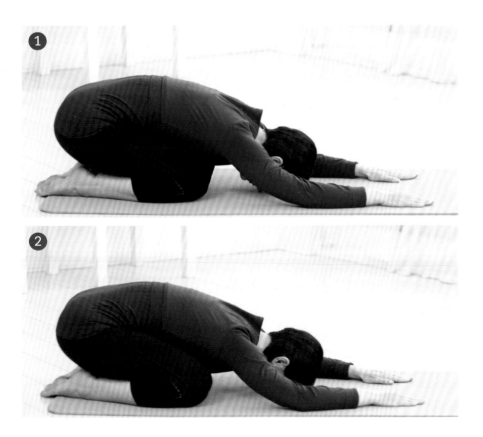

Superman

1. Begin on all-fours, hands under your shoulders, knees directly under your hips and pelvis in neutral. Your back is flat and your neck long (remember the triangle, page 73).

2. Inhale to prepare. Exhale, connect and extend your opposite arm and leg away in a slow controlled movement. Hold for 2 seconds, lengthening the spine from the top of your head to your tailbone. Inhale as you return to the start position, then change sides.

REPEAT 8 TIMES ON EACH SIDE.

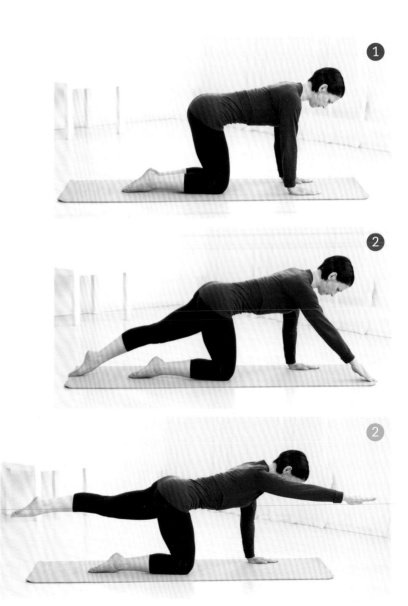

Leg Extensions on All-fours

1. Again begin on all-fours, hands under shoulders, knees directly under your hips and pelvis in neutral. Your back is flat and your neck long (remember the triangle, page 73).

2. Inhale and straighten your left leg behind you, toes still touching the mat.

3. As you exhale, connect and lift your left leg. Gently pulse up and down squeezing the glut muscles, for 12 counts. Inhale as you lower and change leg.

REPEAT 6 TIMES ON EACH LEG.

4. Now when you lift your leg, bend at the knee. Flex your foot and as you exhale, connect and lift towards the ceiling.

REPEAT 12 TIMES.

Then repeat once more, pulsing at the top of the movement 12 times.

REPEAT WITH THE OTHER LEG.

Push back on to your heels into the Shell Stretch (page 95) to give your arms, shoulders and back a nice stretch.

NOTE
– Be careful not to lift your leg too high, rotating the hip and arching the back – the pelvis should remain in neutral.

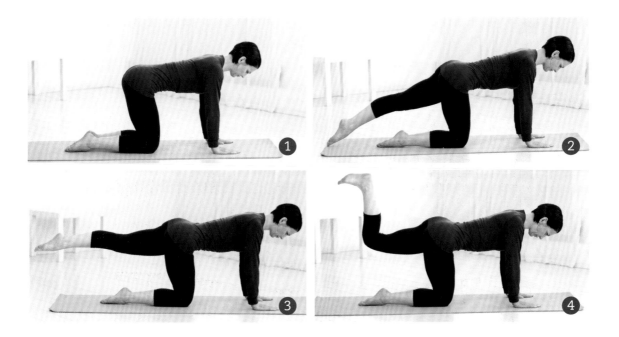

Lower Body Conditioning

The basic set-up for this series of exercises is as follows (if any other modifications are required, I'll let you know). Lie on your side, resting your head on your hand, and place your other hand just in front of your tummy. Keep your chest lifted, navel-to-spine connection 60%, and your hips and shoulders stacked one on top of the other. Now lift your legs and bring them forward to 45 degrees and slightly bend the lower leg to help with stability.

When doing the side leg series, complete all the exercises on one side before you change to the other side.

You are now ready to begin...

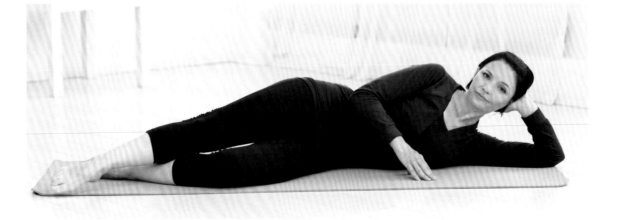

Big Kick

1. Lie on your side in the basic set-up position.

2. Breathe in to prepare and as you exhale, connect and lift your leg with the foot facing upwards to the ceiling.

3. Flex the foot at the top.

4. Inhale as you bring your leg back down to the starting position.

REPEAT 8 TIMES ON EACH SIDE.

NOTE
– *During this exercise make sure you don't arch your back. Just kick your leg as far as you can in a controlled manner without losing your positioning.*

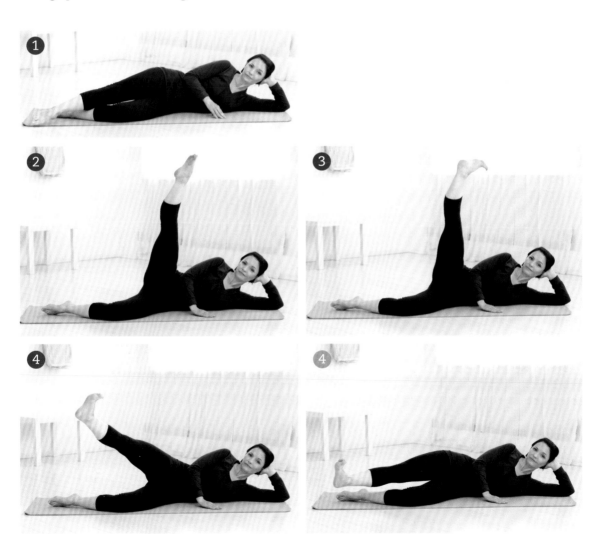

Circles

1. Begin in the basic set-up position.

2. Lift your top leg and draw 8 small circles in each direction, from the hip; then draw 8 big circles in each direction.

3. The toes are pointed and the ankle is static. Remember to keep drawing in your connection throughout and breathe naturally.

REPEAT ON THE OTHER SIDE.

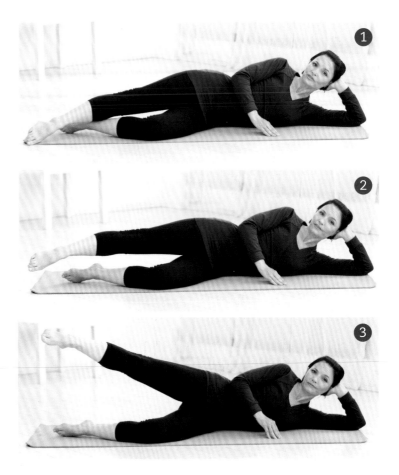

Knee Lifts

1. Begin in the basic set-up position. Now bend both legs and bring them forward to 90 degrees.

2. Breathe in to prepare and as you exhale, connect and lift your upper leg for 2 counts. Then lower it for 2 counts as you inhale.

REPEAT 8 TIMES.

Then lift your leg up and down for 8 single counts, so this time a bit faster.

REPEAT ON THE OTHER SIDE.

NOTE
– Perform this exercise at a steady pace and don't rest your upper leg on your lower leg in-between the repetitions.
– Remember to keep the chest lifted and the abdominals drawn in.

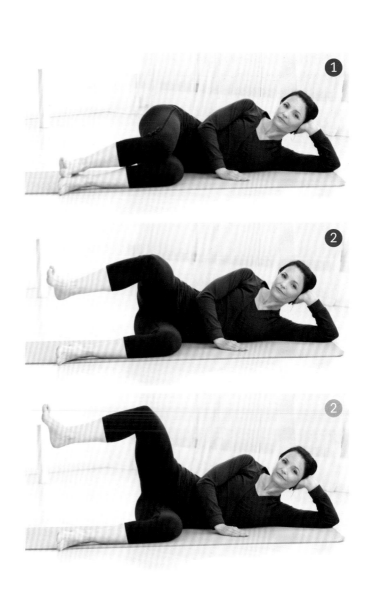

Kick Kick Forward

1. Begin in the basic set-up position then bring your lower leg forward to 90 degrees.

2. Breathe in to prepare. On the exhale, connect, flex your top foot and kick forward in a 'one, two' beat at the end of the kick to stretch out your hamstring.

3. Point your toe as you return the leg and stretch through the front of the hip flexor and thigh.

REPEAT 8 TIMES ON EACH SIDE.

NOTE
– Kick only as far as is comfortable for you, being careful not to arch your back and lose the basic set-up position.

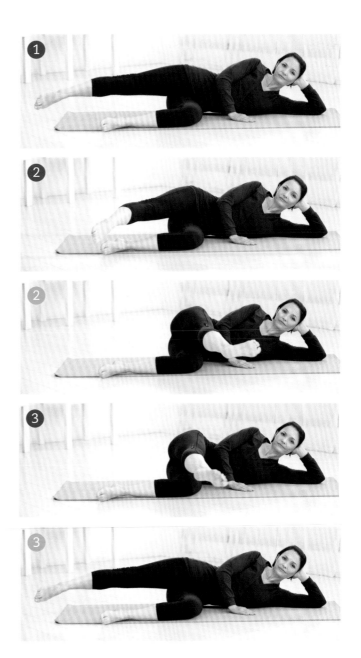

Clams

1. Begin in the basic set-up position. Bend the upper leg, place it over the lower leg and line your heels up with your bottom. Lift the heels and tilt the hips slightly forward.

2. Breathe in to prepare. Exhale, connect and, keeping your feet together, raise your top knee to open the clam for a count of 2, and close it for a count of 2 as you breathe in again.

Repeat 8 times and then open and close your knee on single counts for 8. Now hold the clam open and finish with 8 pulses.

REPEAT ON THE OTHER SIDE.

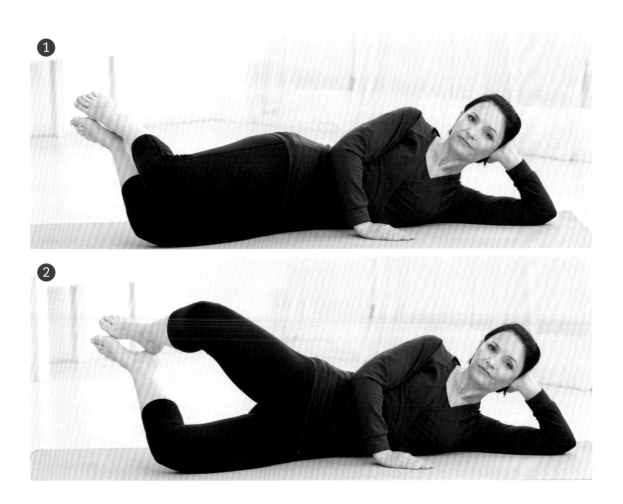

Bananas

1. Lie on your side and create a banana-shaped curve with the full length of your body, both legs extended and arms stretched above your head, palms together.

2. Breathe in to prepare. Exhale, connect and bring your upper arm up over your head to the front of your thigh while lifting both legs about 6 inches off the mat. Press gently through your lower elbow as you lift. Reverse the movement back to the start position as you breathe in.

REPEAT 8 TIMES ON EACH SIDE.

NOTE
– When you return to the start position, always drop your head down rather than trying to hold it up in-between the movements, which will give you a sore neck.

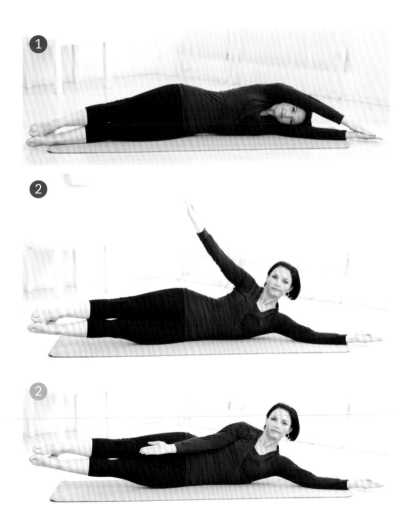

Inner Thigh Lifts

1. Sit on the mat with your knees bent. Rest back on to your elbows, but don't let your body sink into the mat. Keep the chest lifted. Extend one leg in front of you and take it out to a 45 degree angle. Rotate the leg slightly out from the hip and flex the foot.

2. Breathe in to prepare and as you exhale, connect and lift the leg for a count of 2 diagonally to the opposite knee. Breathe in as you lower back down for a count of 2.

REPEAT 10 TIMES ON EACH SIDE.

NOTE
– You should really feel this in your inner thigh. If not, check that you are rotating the leg from your hip and flexing your foot before your lift.

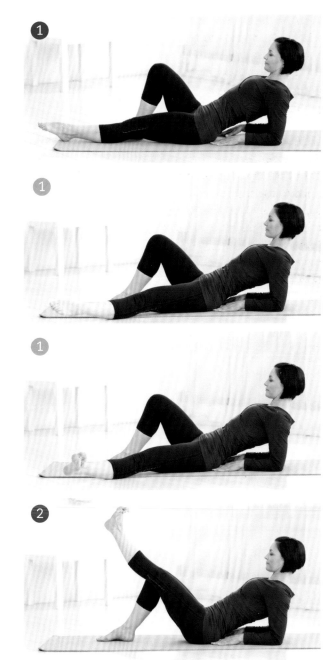

Squats

1. Stand with your feet hip-width apart, arms by your sides.

2. Imagine you are going to sit back on to a chair. Breathe in as you squat down, keeping your back straight, arms extended and knees behind your toes. Exhale and connect as you push back up through your heels to the start position.

REPEAT 12 TIMES.

3. Now squat down deeper and hold the squat at the bottom of the move for a count of 2 before pushing back up.

REPEAT 12 TIMES.

4. Finally, take your feet slightly wider and place your hands on your hips. Squat down and push through your toes as you explode back up.

REPEAT 12 TIMES.

NOTE
– *Keep your shoulders relaxed and don't let your knees drift forward beyond your toes while performing the squats.*
– *Remember to maintain your connection throughout to protect your lower back.*
– *If you experience discomfort in the lower back, don't squat so low. Also check that you are still drawing in your connection. Once you get the hang of the movement, you can always try deepening the squat again.*

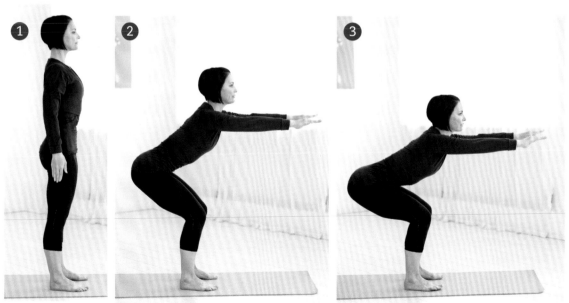

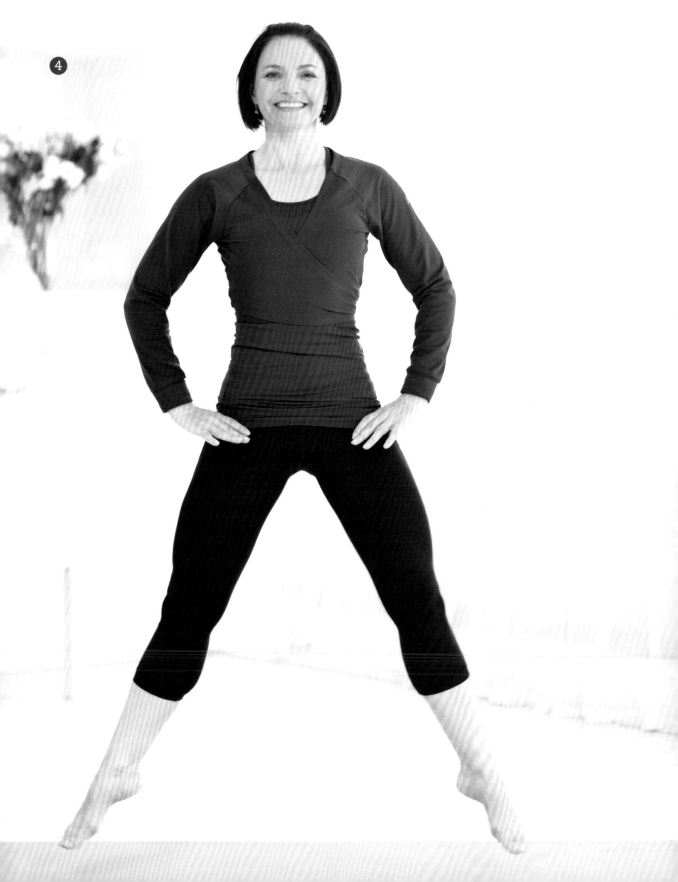

Adductor Squats

1. Take your feet out wide to the sides, turning them out slightly, and rest your hands on the tops of your thighs.

2. Breathe in and squat down for a count of 2. As you exhale, connect and push up for a count of 2 through your heels, working your inner thighs and bottom.

REPEAT 12 TIMES.

Now drop down again and pulse at the bottom of the squat for a count of 12.

NOTE
– Make sure you keep your connection strong throughout to prevent any discomfort in the lower back, and keep your knees directly over your heels.

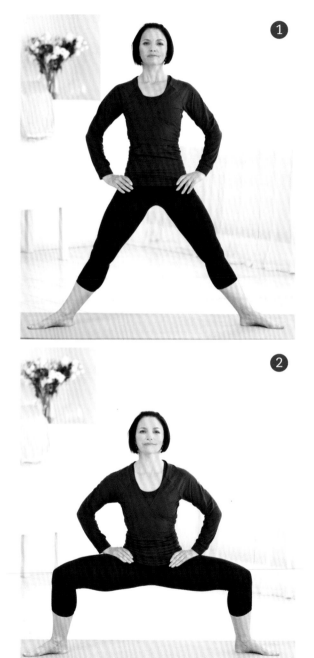

Lunges

1. Stand with your feet hip-width apart, hands on hips.

2. Take a big step forward with your left leg. Allow the right heel to lift so you are resting on the ball of your right foot. Keep your feet hip-width apart.

3. Breathe in, tuck your tailbone under and gently drop down. Exhale, connect and push straight back up to the start position.

REPEAT 12 TIMES ON ONE LEG; THEN PULSE FOR 12 AT THE BOTTOM OF THE LAST LUNGE BEFORE SWAPPING TO THE OTHER LEG.

NOTE
– Make sure your front knee remains behind your toe and your feet are hip-width apart. Check that your shoulders are directly above your hips and your back knee is directly below your hip.
– Make sure that you don't push forward while lunging, but perform a simple up and down motion using your bottom and legs.

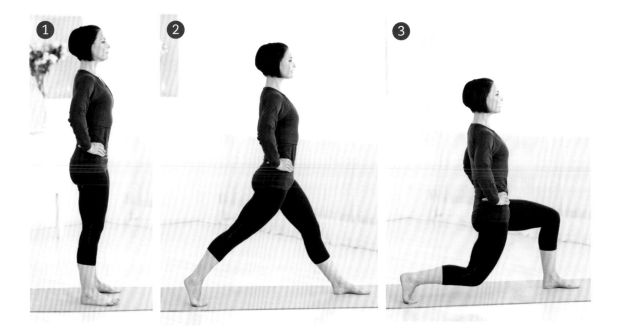

20 minute workout

For this final section, I've put together a routine that builds on the Pilates moves you've learned, but with faster-paced repetitions, designed to raise your heart rate and really sculpt and tone your body.

SQUATS (PAGE 106)

Breathe in as you squat down, exhale and connect as you push back up through your heels. **REPEAT 12 TIMES.**

Squat down and hold at the bottom for a count of 2 before pushing back up. **REPEAT 12 TIMES.**

Take your feet slightly wider and place your hands on your thighs. Squat down and push through your toes as you explode back up to the start position. **REPEAT 12 TIMES.**

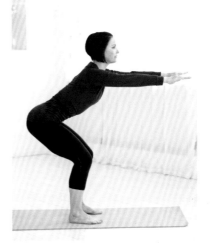

LUNGES (PAGE 109)

Take a big step forward, tuck your tailbone under and gently drop down. Exhale, connect and push straight back up. **REPEAT 12 TIMES ON ONE LEG, PULSING AT THE BOTTOM OF THE LAST ONE FOR 12 BEFORE PUSHING BACK UP. REPEAT ON THE OTHER LEG.**

From a standing position, gently drop your head and roll your spine downwards and then walk your hands out along the mat in front of you into the Full Press-up position. Drop the knees on to the mat if you prefer to do a Half Press-up.

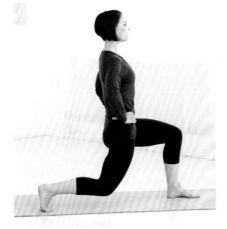

PRESS-UPS (PAGE 73)

Inhale and draw your tummy in 100%, keeping your body taut and in a straight line as you descend. Exhale as you push back up. **REPEAT 5 TIMES.**

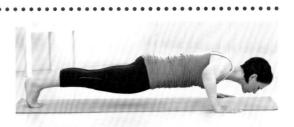

DART WITH ARM BEATS
(PAGE 82)

Lift your head, shoulders, hands and feet off the mat and beat both hands towards the centre of your back for 10 beats, using short exhales. REPEAT 8 TIMES WITH 10 HAND BEATS, RESTING IN-BETWEEN.

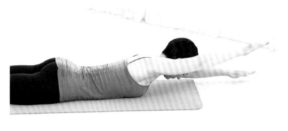

SWIMMING (PAGE 83)

Use short exhales to raise opposite arms and legs alternately in a swimming motion. COMPLETE 3 SETS OF 16 COUNTS, RESTING IN-BETWEEN.

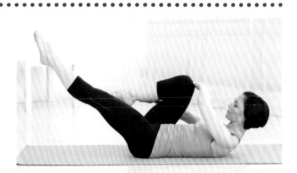

SINGLE LEG STRETCH
(PAGE 63)

With an imprinted spine and knees in table-top position, lift your head and shoulders and bring alternate knees towards your chest, extending the other leg at the same time. Tap one hand to the outside of the ankle on the bent leg and the other to the top of this knee. REPEAT SLOWLY 12 TIMES ON EACH LEG.

CRISS CROSS (PAGE 65)

Spine imprinted, rotate your upper body, lifting your right shoulder to meet your left knee, and then repeat on the other side, lowering your upper body (including your head) completely to the mat between each movement. REPEAT SLOWLY 12 TIMES ON EACH SIDE.

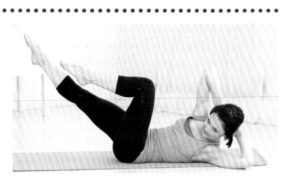

DOUBLE LEG STRETCH
(PAGE 68)

Knees in table-top position, head and shoulders lifted, hands lifted to either side of the knees. Extend your arms back to the side of the ears and extend your legs away from the body, keeping toes pointed and back imprinted on the mat. Slowly circle your arms back to the side of the legs and return the legs to table-top position.
REPEAT 8 TIMES.

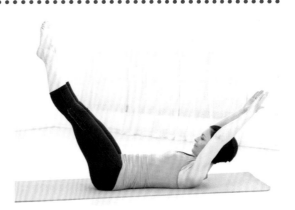

SINGLE STRAIGHT LEG STRETCH (PAGE 64)

Spine imprinted, extend both legs towards the ceiling, toes pointed, head and shoulders lifted. Pull one leg towards you and lower the other away, pulsing for 2 quick beats.
REPEAT 12 TIMES ON EACH LEG.

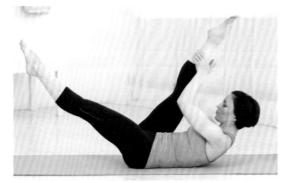

ROLL-UP WITH A TWIST
(PAGE 69)

Curl the upper body off the mat one vertebra at a time to 90 degrees, keeping your shoulders back and down; slowly twist from the waist to one side and then the other, before rolling back down. **REPEAT 8 TIMES.**

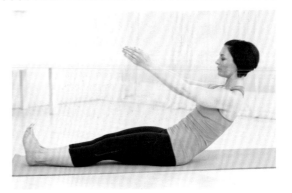

LONG BODY STRETCH
(PAGE 71)

Stretch your whole body, extending the tips of your fingers and toes, then relax. Stretch just the right side, then the left; finally, slightly arch your ribcage to stretch the front of your abdominals.

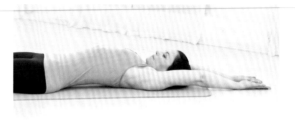

KNEE LIFTS (PAGE 101)

Begin in the basic set-up position. Now bend both legs and bring them forward to 90 degrees. Breathe in to prepare and as you exhale, connect and lift your upper leg for 2 counts. Then lower it for 2 counts as you inhale. REPEAT 8 TIMES ON EACH SIDE. Then lift your leg up and down for single counts, so this time a bit faster. REPEAT 8 TIMES ON EACH SIDE.

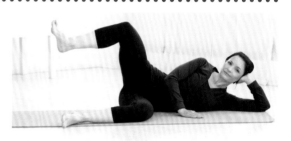

CIRCLES (PAGE 100)

Begin in the basic set-up position. Lift your top leg and draw 8 small circles in each direction, from the hip; then draw 8 big circles in each direction.

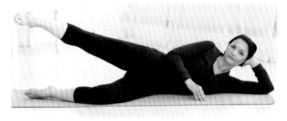

CLAMS (PAGE 103)

Lie on your side in the clam position, raise your upper leg for a count of 2, then close for a count of 2. REPEAT 12 TIMES. On the last one, hold the clam open and pulse for 12. REPEAT ON THE OTHER SIDE.

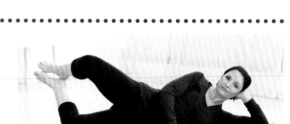

BANANAS (PAGE 104)

Create a banana-shaped curve with the full length of your body, then bring your upper arm up over your head to the front of your thigh while lifting both legs about 6 inches off the mat. Press gently through your lower elbow as you lift. REPEAT 12 TIMES ON EACH SIDE, REVERSING THE MOVEMENT BACK TO THE START POSITION EACH TIME.

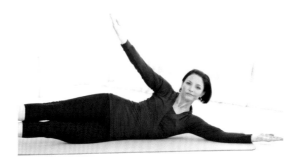

INNER THIGH LIFTS (PAGE 105)

Rest back on to your elbows, extend one leg out in front of you and take it out to a 45 degree angle. Rotate the leg slightly out from the hip and flex the foot. Lift the leg for a count of 2 diagonally towards the opposite knee. Then lower back down. REPEAT 10 TIMES ON EACH SIDE.

Finish by slowly rolling up to a seated position one vertebra at a time, keeping your shoulders back and down.

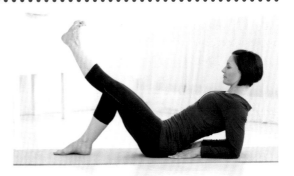

Cool down

We're now going to spend some time stretching and relaxing your body, cooling down after the workout and getting you ready for the rest of your day.

Long Body Stretch

1. Lie on your back, legs lengthened along the mat, arms above your head and shoulders relaxed.

2. Breathe in, and as you exhale stretch your whole body, extending the tips of your fingers and toes; then relax. Inhale again and stretch only the right side of the body as you exhale – remember to stretch the fingers and toes. Repeat on the left side.

3. Finally, stretch the whole body again, but this time slightly arch your ribcage   to stretch the front of your abdominals. Hold each stretch for the duration of the breath.

Roll up as you prepare for Spine Stretch.

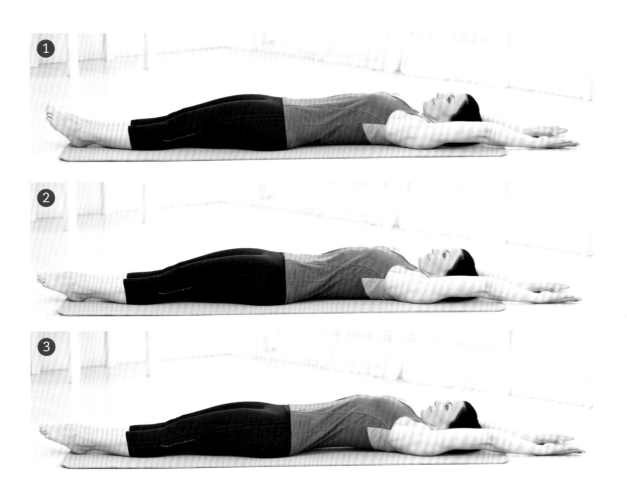

Spine Stretch

1. Sit in a neutral spine position, legs straight and opened slightly wider than your hips. Extend your arms in front of you level with the shoulders, palms facing towards the centre. Feet should be flexed. Try not to collapse in the upper body – imagine you are being pulled up by a thread through the top of your head. Inhale to prepare.

2. Exhale, connect and drop your head forward between your arms. Then extend forward with your arms to stretch through the upper back. Simultaneously, as you stretch the upper back, imagine someone is pulling you backwards from the waist stretching your lower back. Inhale, and on the exhale return to the start position.

REPEAT 3 TIMES.

Roll down on to the mat as you prepare for a Lower Back, Chest and Shoulder Stretch.

NOTE
– *Remember to maintain the navel-to-spine connection throughout this exercise to protect the lower back.*
– *For comfort you may want to sit on a small cushion while doing this exercise. This will keep the pelvis at the right angle and relieve any discomfort on the back of the legs.*

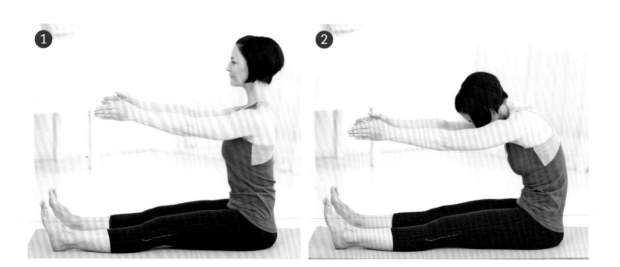

Lower Back, Chest and Shoulder Stretch

1. Begin on the mat in a neutral spine position and lengthen the right leg. Draw the left knee up, then take it across the right leg, keeping a 90 degree angle at the back of the knee. Keep both shoulders on the mat and gently turn your head in the opposite direction. Place the right hand on the left knee and take the left hand (palm facing up) out to the side of the body just below shoulder height.

2. Breathe in, and as you exhale, connect and press gently on the left knee, stretching through the lower back while stretching the left hand away and opening the chest and shoulder.

REPEAT 3 TIMES ON EACH SIDE, HOLDING EACH STRETCH FOR THE DURATION OF THE BREATH.

Come back to a neutral spine position as you prepare for a Glute Stretch.

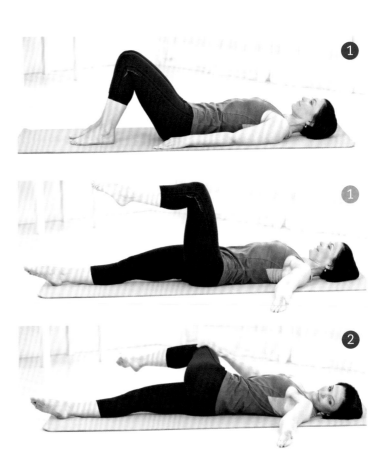

Glute Stretch

1. Begin in a neutral spine position. Draw the right knee into your chest and place your right ankle on top of your left thigh. Inhale to prepare.

2. Exhale, connect and lift the head and left leg and inter-lace both hands around the back of the left thigh. Then drop your head back down on the mat. Breathe in and as you exhale draw the left thigh towards the chest feeling a stretch in the right glute.

REPEAT 3 TIMES ON EACH SIDE, HOLDING EACH STRETCH FOR THE DURATION OF THE BREATH.

Now roll over to prepare for a Quad Stretch.

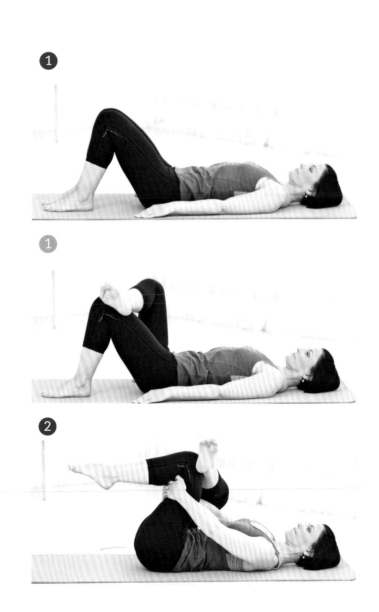

Quad Stretch

1. Lie on your front, head resting on the back of your hands.

2. Inhale, bend your right knee and take hold of the foot with your right hand. Exhale, connect and pull the foot towards your bottom to feel a stretch down the front of your leg. Keep your pelvis on the mat throughout the stretch.

REPEAT 3 TIMES ON EACH SIDE AND HOLD EACH STRETCH FOR THE DURATION OF THE BREATH.

Push back to prepare for the Kitty Cat.

NOTE
– If you experience any discomfort in the lower back, place a small pillow under the stomach.

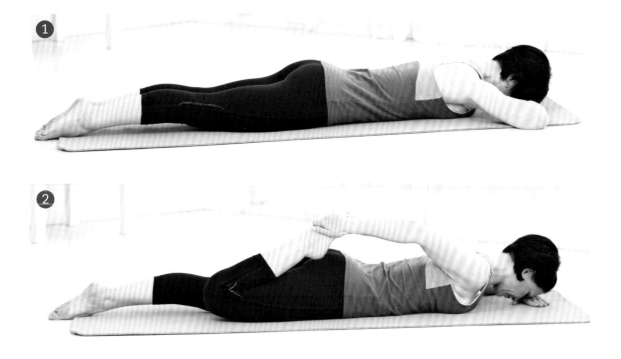

The Kitty Cat

1. Begin on all-fours, your hands slightly wider than your shoulders, your knees directly under your hips and your pelvis in neutral. Your back is flat and your neck long (remember the triangle, page 73). Inhale to prepare.

2. As you exhale, connect and drop your head forward, arch the upper back and feel your tailbone tucking under.

3. Move your bottom back towards your heels, feeling a stretch through the spine.

4. Inhale as you bend the elbows out to the sides and skim your nose along the mat until your face passes through your hands.

5. Then exhale, drop your head, push up and arch the upper back as you begin again.

REPEAT 6 TIMES.

Sit back on your heels to prepare for a Chest and Shoulder Stretch.

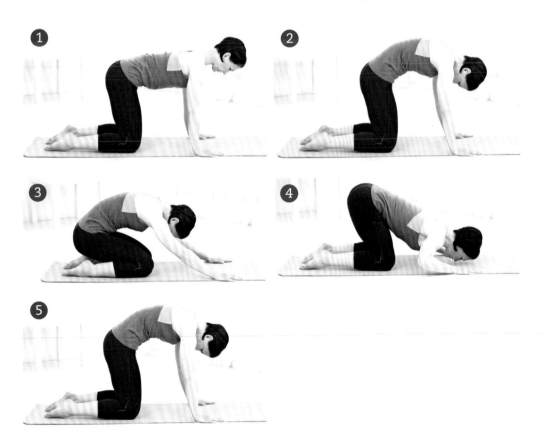

Chest and Shoulder Stretch

1. Sit on your heels looking straight ahead with your chest high and palms resting on the front of the legs.

2. Breathe in, and as you exhale, connect and extend your arms to the sides to open and stretch the front of your chest and shoulders.

REPEAT 3 TIMES AND HOLD FOR THE DURATION OF THE BREATH.

Now go on to all-fours to prepare for the Downward Dog.

NOTE
– If sitting on your heels is uncomfortable, stand on the knees to complete the stretch.

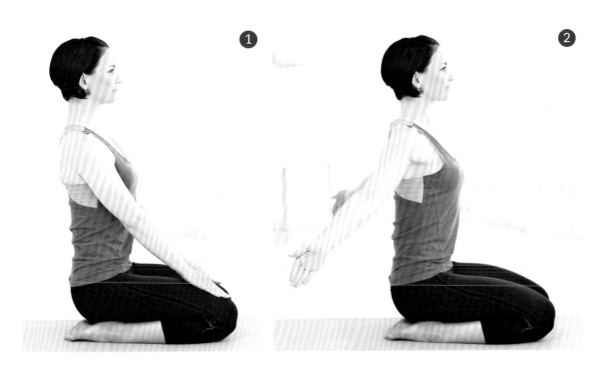

Downward Dog

1. Begin on all-fours, your hands under your shoulders, your knees directly under your hips and your pelvis in neutral. Your back is flat and your neck long (remember the triangle, page 73).

2. Inhale, drop your head forward and tuck your toes under. Exhale, connect and press up and back through the heel of your hands to stretch the shoulders and lengthen through the back.

3. Inhale again, and as you exhale drop your heels, raising your hips higher as you continue to push through the heel of your hands to stretch your hamstrings and calves. The head remains positioned between your arms so that you are looking at your feet and keeping your back long. Inhale into the mid back and soften the knees to release the stretch.

As you exhale again, connect and press back up to stretch, checking there is no tension in the neck or shoulders.

REPEAT 3 TIMES, HOLDING FOR 3 DEEP BREATHS EACH TIME.

Inhale and walk your hands in towards your feet, exhale, connect and gently roll up to standing, stacking the vertebrae one by one and rolling the shoulders back and down.

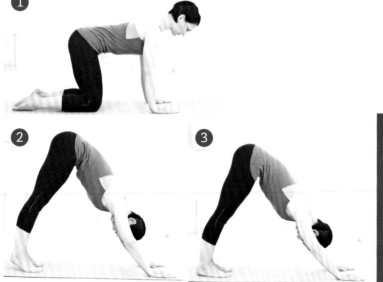

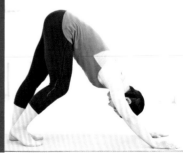

> **VARIATION**
> *Also try bending at the knee and stretching through one leg at a time.*

Hamstring Stretch

1. Open your legs slightly wider than your hips and extend both arms out to 45 degrees.

2. Breathe in to prepare. Exhale, connect and flex forward from the hips to 90 degrees, keeping your back flat, chest high and neck lengthened.

Inhale, then exhale and bring your weight forward on to your toes, and feel the stretch through the back of the legs.

HOLD FOR 3 BREATHS, STRETCHING DEEPER ON EACH EXHALATION.

Come back up and take your feet wider for your Adductor Stretch.

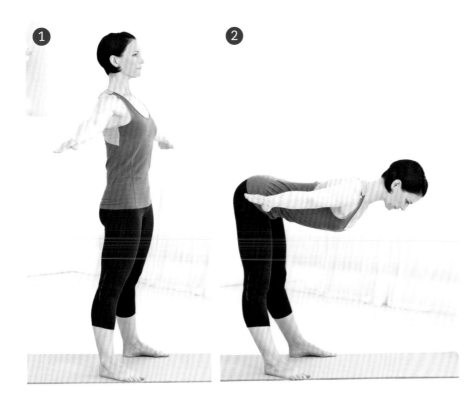

Adductor Stretch

1. Open your legs considerably wider than your hips and extend both arms to 90 degrees. Your heels should be positioned directly under your palms.

2. Bend one knee out to the side and keep the other leg straight, turning the foot on this leg forward. Place both hands on your knee. Breathe in, and as you exhale, connect and drop the body closer to the bent knee, feeling a stretch all the way along the inside of the extended leg.

REPEAT 3 TIMES ON EACH LEG, HOLDING EACH STRETCH FOR THE DURATION OF THE BREATH.

Release the stretch during the inhale by straightening the knee for a few seconds.

Then walk your feet in and roll up to standing for a Side Stretch.

NOTE
– *Ensure the knee remains above the heel when you perform this stretch.*

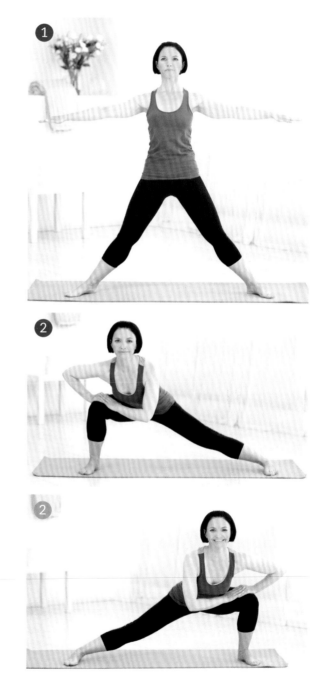

Side Stretch

1. Begin by crossing your left foot over your right foot. Then extend your left arm up to the side of your head, palm facing forward.

2. Breathe in, and as you exhale, connect and stretch up and over to the right, feeling the stretch all the way along your side. Inhale and come back to the centre.

REPEAT 3 TIMES ON EACH SIDE, HOLDING EACH STRETCH FOR THE DURATION OF THE BREATH.

Now, separate the feet for some final twisting and breathing.

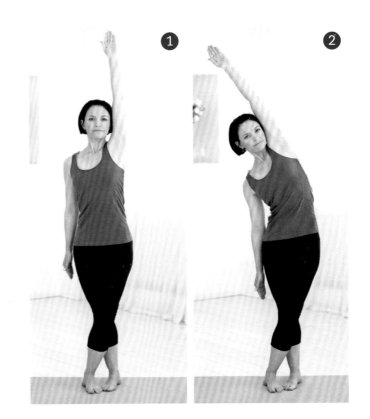

Twist to Wake Up the Body

1. Stand tall, feet slightly wider than hip-width apart, arms extended 45 degrees, spine lengthened and upper body relaxed.

2. Breathe in to prepare and as you exhale, connect and start to rotate around the spine, moving from the waist, allowing the arms and legs to follow.

REPEAT 10 TIMES ROTATING FROM SIDE TO SIDE.

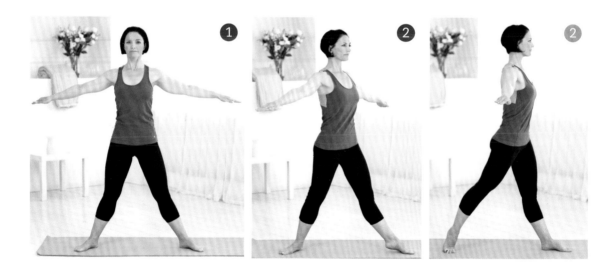

Breathing

1. Begin with your feet considerably wider than your hips and slightly turned out.Inhale as you bend your knees out to the side and drop the body down, arms crossed in front of the chest.

2. Exhale, and connect as you push up through the heels, straightening the legs and circling the arms out to the sides and above the head.

3. Inhale as you circle the arms down again, bringing them back across your chest while lowering the body ready to start again.

REPEAT 6 TIMES, TAKING DEEP BREATHS.

Pilates is for life, so take what you've learned in this workout – breathing, exhaling on the effort, and drawing in your navel-to-spine connection whenever effort is required – into your everyday life!

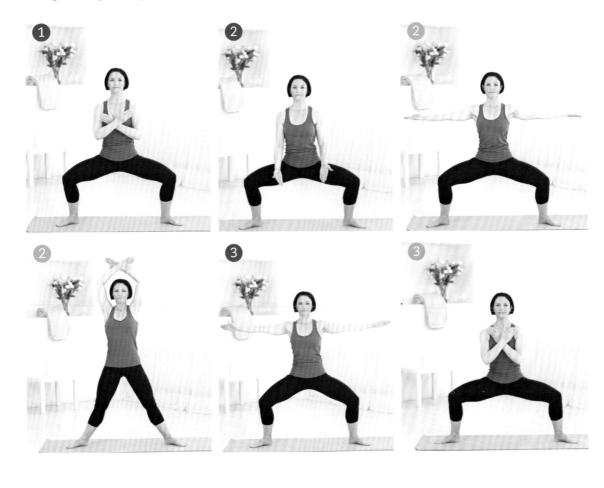

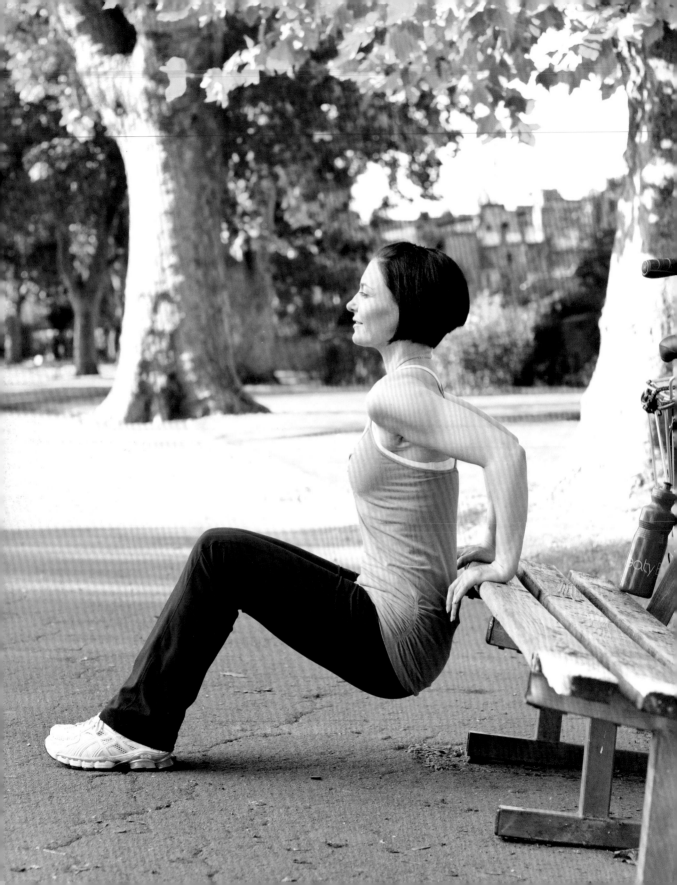

'I have to exercise in the morning before my brain figures out what I'm doing.' Marsha

Pilates on the go

This little routine is perfect for rolling out of bed and waking up your body and mind first thing. It will put a spring in your step and gently tone your body at the same time.

5 Minutes
in the Morning

LATERAL BREATHING
(PAGE 44)

To begin, lie on your back with your knees bent at 90 degrees, your arms by your sides, plams facing upwards. Breathe in slowly for a count of 5 and exhale for 10, building your 60% connection. Keep your pelvis in neutral placement (see page 42) and your body relaxed.

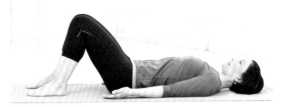

PELVIC PEELING (PAGE 53)

From a neutral spine position, tilt the pelvis, gently press the lower back to the mat, then peel one vertebra at a time off the mat up to the mid back, creating a straight line with your body. **RAISE AND LOWER 6 TIMES.**

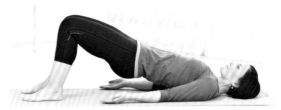

HIP ROLLS (PAGE 54)

Lie in a neutral spine position, arms extended out to the sides just below shoulder level, and roll your knees to the side (keeping your feet together and both shoulders on the mat) while turning your head in the opposite direction. **REPEAT 6 TIMES ON EACH SIDE.**

LONG BODY STRETCH
(PAGE 57)

Stretch your whole body, extending the tips of your fingers and toes, then relax. Stretch just the right side, then the left; finally, slightly arch your ribcage to stretch the front of your abdominals.

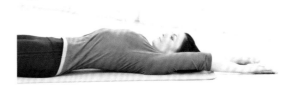

SINGLE LEG STRETCH
(PAGE 63)

With an imprinted spine and knees in table-top position, lift your head and shoulders and bring alternate knees towards your chest, extending the other leg at the same time. Tap one hand to the outside of the ankle on the bent leg and the other to the top of this knee. **REPEAT SLOWLY 12 TIMES ON EACH LEG.**

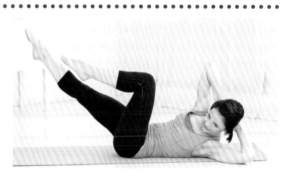

CRISS CROSS (PAGE 65)

Spine imprinted, rotate your upper body, lifting your right shoulder to meet your left knee, and then repeat on the other side, lowering your upper body (including your head) completely to the mat between each movement. **REPEAT SLOWLY 12 TIMES ON EACH SIDE.**

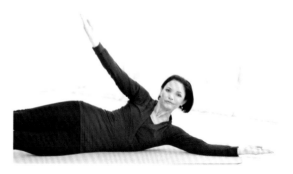

BANANAS (PAGE 104)

Create a banana-shaped curve with the full length of your body, then bring your upper arm up over your head to the front of your thigh while lifting both legs about 6 inches off the mat. Press gently through your lower elbow as you lift. **REPEAT 12 TIMES ON EACH SIDE, REVERSING THE MOVEMENT BACK TO THE START EACH TIME.**

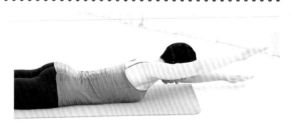

SWIMMING (PAGE 83)

Use short exhales to raise opposite arms and legs alternately in a swimming motion. **COMPLETE 3 SETS OF 16 COUNTS, RESTING IN-BETWEEN.**

PRESS-UPS (PAGE 73)

Draw in a 100% connection, keeping your body taut and in a straight line as you descend. Exhale as you push back up, pressing through your palms. Choose Box, Half or Full Press-ups (or a mixture of all 3). **TRY TO COMPLETE 12.**

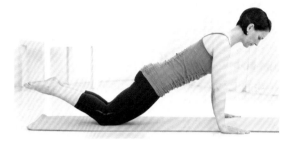

THE KITTY CAT (PAGE 84)

On all-fours, slowly curl your spine up and then back, lowering your bottom before you scoop down and forwards, and finally back up to the start position. **REPEAT SLOWLY 6 TIMES.**

Roll-up to a standing position.

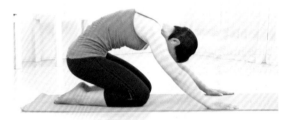

SQUATS (PAGE 106)

Breathe in as you squat down, keeping your back straight, arms extended and knees behind your toes. Exhale and connect as you push back up through your heels to the start position. **REPEAT SLOWLY 12 TIMES.**

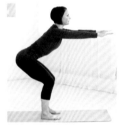

TWIST TO WAKE UP THE BODY (PAGE 128)

Stand tall, feet slightly wider than hip-width apart, arms extended 45 degrees, spine lengthened and upper body relaxed. Breathe in to prepare and as you exhale, connect and start to rotate around the spine, moving from the waist, allowing the arms and legs to follow. **REPEAT 10 TIMES ROTATING FROM SIDE TO SIDE.**

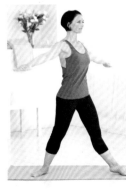

In the Zone:
5 Minute Abs 1

From a standing position, gently lower the head and begin by rolling down through the spine to the mat, one vertebra at a time. Take a deep breath at the bottom, then begin to come back up, stacking the vertebrae as you roll back up to standing. **REPEAT SLOWLY 3 TIMES.**

HEEL DROPS (PAGE 60)

Spine imprinted and knees in table-top position, exhale and connect as you flex from the hip, moving the heel slowly towards the mat; then come back to table-top position. **REPEAT SLOWLY 12 TIMES ON EACH SIDE.**

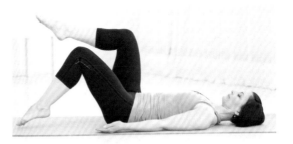

LEG EXTENSIONS (PAGE 61)

Spine imprinted and knees in table-top position, cradle your head in your hands and lift. Extend one leg to a 45 degree angle; then draw back to table-top position. **REPEAT SLOWLY 12 TIMES ON EACH SIDE, ALTERNATING AND KEEPING EACH LEG EXTENDED FOR 2 SECONDS.**

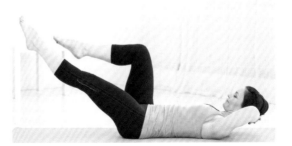

SINGLE LEG STRETCH
(PAGE 63)

With an imprinted spine and knees in table-top position, lift your head and shoulders and bring alternate knees towards your chest, extending the other leg at the same time. Tap one hand to the outside of the ankle on the bent leg and the other to the top of this knee. **REPEAT SLOWLY 12 TIMES ON EACH LEG.**

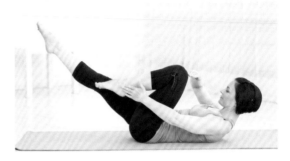

CRISS CROSS (PAGE 65)

Spine imprinted, rotate your upper body, lifting your right shoulder to meet your left knee, and then repeat on the other side, lowering your upper body (including your head) completely to the mat between each movement. **REPEAT SLOWLY 12 TIMES ON EACH SIDE.**

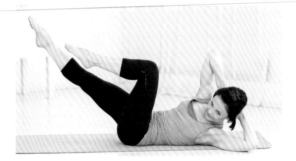

PARALLEL ABDOMINALS
(PAGE 67)

Spine imprinted and knees in table-top position, arms extended above the chest, palms facing down. Inhale to prepare and as you exhale, connect and slowly press your arms to the sides of your body (imagine you are pushing through treacle) while lifting your head and extending your legs, lowering them 6 to 12 inches away from your body, in one gentle fluid movement. Inhale and slowly reverse the movement, bringing the body back to the start position. **REPEAT SLOWLY 8 TIMES.**

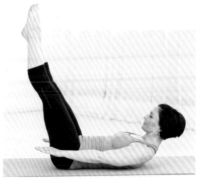

BANANAS (PAGE 104)

Create a banana-shaped curve with the full length of your body, then bring your upper arm up over your head to the front of your thigh while lifting both legs about 6 inches off the mat. Press gently through your lower elbow as you lift. **REPEAT 12 TIMES ON EACH SIDE, REVERSING THE MOVEMENT BACK TO THE START EACH TIME.**

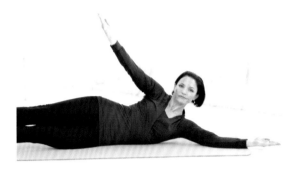

LONG BODY STRETCH
(PAGE 57)

Stretch your whole body, extending the tips of your fingers and toes, then relax. Stretch just the right side, then the left; finally, slightly arch your ribcage to stretch the front of your abdominals.

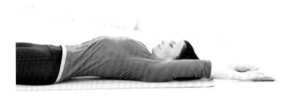

'Like all brides, I wanted to look as fabulous as I could for my wedding day and so I enlisted Margot's help for getting into the best shape of my life in time for the big day. I knew my arms and shoulders would be on show, so as well as toning my tummy, because who doesn't want a flat tummy, Margot gave me some fantastic exercises I could easily practise at home for giving my arms definition and tone for the first time since I could remember! As a result of Pilates, my posture really improved to give my shoulders a lovely line and I felt so confident as I walked down the aisle. Other exercises make you fit, but Pilates gave me such a lovely shape, toned but still very feminine.' Aileen

In the Zone:
5 Minute Abs 2

From a standing position, gently lower the head and begin by rolling down through the spine to the mat, one vertebra at a time. Take a deep breath at the bottom, then begin to come back up, stacking the vertebrae as you roll back up to standing. **REPEAT SLOWLY 3 TIMES.**

SINGLE LEG STRETCH
(PAGE 63)

With an imprinted spine and knees in table-top position, lift your head and shoulders and bring alternate knees towards your chest, extending the other leg at the same time. Tap one hand to the outside of the ankle on the bent leg and the other to the top of this knee. **REPEAT SLOWLY 12 TIMES ON EACH LEG.**

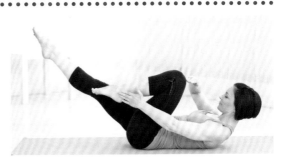

DOUBLE LEG STRETCH
(PAGE 68)

Knees in table-top position, head and shoulders lifted, hands lifted to either side of the knees, extend your arms back to the side of the ears and extend your legs away from the body, keeping toes pointed and back imprinted on the mat. Slowly circle your arms back to the side of the legs and return the legs to table-top position. **REPEAT 12 TIMES.**

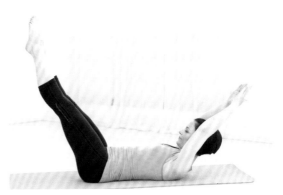

DOUBLE LEG LOWER
AND LIFT (PAGE 66)

Spine imprinted, knees in table-top position, extend both legs towards the ceiling, toes pointed. Lift the head and slowly lower the legs 6 to 12 inches; then turn out your legs from the hips and flex your feet before drawing the legs back up to centre. **REPEAT SLOWLY 12 TIMES.**

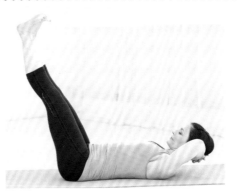

CRISS CROSS (PAGE 65)

Spine imprinted, rotate your upper body, lifting your right shoulder to meet your left knee, and then repeat on the other side, lowering your upper body (including your head) completely to the mat between each movement. **REPEAT SLOWLY 12 TIMES ON EACH SIDE.**

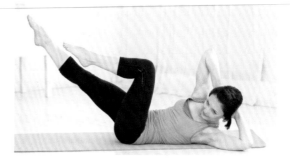

THE HUNDRED (PAGE 62)

Spine imprinted, knees in table-top position, curl your head and shoulders off the mat and pump your arms up and down 100 times – imagine you are splashing your arms in water.

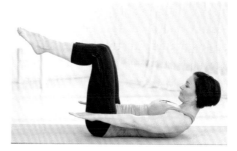

HALF PLANK (PAGE 87)

Begin on all-fours with your hands directly under your shoulders and neck lengthened (remember the triangle, page 73). Extend one knee back followed by the other and lift your feet off the mat. Drop your bottom to create a straight diagonal line with your body. Draw your connection in 100%. Breathe in for a count of 2, and exhale for a count of 2 as you push away from the mat with the heels of your hands. **HOLD THE POSITION FOR 2 LOTS OF 30 SECONDS.**

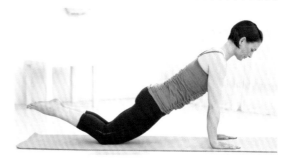

FULL PLANK (PAGE 88)

From the Half Plank position, tuck your toes under and lift your knees to create a long diagonal line with your whole body. Remember to keep 100% connection and lengthen the neck. Breathe in for a count of 2 and out for a count of 2, pressing away from the mat with the heels of your hands. **HOLD FOR 2 LOTS OF 30 SECONDS.**

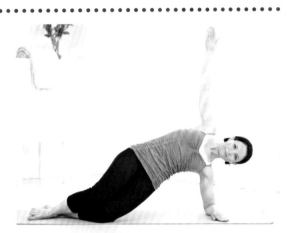

SIDE PLANK (PAGE 89)

Turn on to your side, bending your knees at 90 degrees and resting on your elbow, which should be positioned directly under your shoulder. Split your feet so that your top foot is on the mat, just ahead of your bottom foot; this will give you better balance. With legs still bent, breathe in to prepare. Exhale, connect 100% and lift your body up, raising the top arm straight up. Hold for 30 seconds. Reverse the movement back to the start position as you breathe in. **REPEAT TWICE ON EACH SIDE.**

THE KITTY CAT (PAGE 84)

On all-fours, slowly curl your spine up and then back, lowering your bottom before you scoop down and forwards, and finally back up to the start position. **REPEAT SLOWLY 6 TIMES.**

From all-fours, tuck your toes under, slowly walk your hands back and begin to roll-up to a standing position.

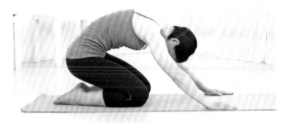

In the Zone:
5 Minute Bottom and Thighs

SQUATS (PAGE 106)

Breathe in as you squat down, exhale and connect as you push back up through your heels. **REPEAT 12 TIMES.**

Take your feet slightly wider and place your hands on your thighs. Squat down and push through your toes as you explode back up to the start position. **REPEAT 12 TIMES.**

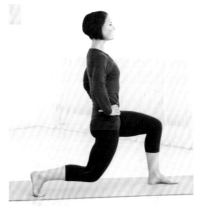

LUNGES (PAGE 109)

Take a big step forward, tuck your tailbone under and gently drop down. Exhale, connect and push straight back up. **REPEAT 12 TIMES ON ONE LEG, THEN SWAP OVER.**

From a standing position, gently drop the head and roll downwards through the spine, then walk your hands out along the mat in front of you, dropping your knees into an all-fours position.

LEG EXTENSIONS ON ALL-FOURS (PAGE 97)

Begin on all-fours, hands under shoulders, knees directly under your hips and pelvis in neutral. Your back is flat and your neck long (remember the triangle, page 73). Inhale and straighten your left leg behind you. Lift and bend at the knee. Flex your foot and as you exhale, connect and lift towards the ceiling. **REPEAT 12 TIMES. THEN REPEAT ONCE MORE, PULSING AT THE TOP OF THE MOVEMENT 12 TIMES. THEN REPEAT WITH THE OTHER LEG.**

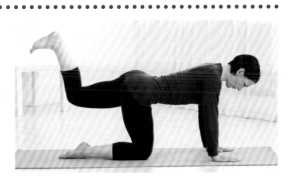

'I've lost 2lb this week and my bum feels as hard as steel… way to go, Margot!' Emma

SHELL STRETCH (PAGE 95)

Push back, rest your bottom on your heels to give your arms, shoulders and back a nice stretch. Do this first with your knees together and then open the knees slightly and let your bottom sink deeper as you exhale.

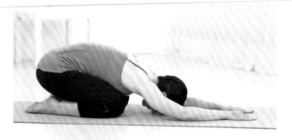

BIG KICK (PAGE 99)

Lie on your side and lift your leg with the foot facing upwards to the ceiling, flex at the top before lowering to start position.
REPEAT 12 TIMES ON EACH SIDE.

Note: Complete all the side leg exercises on one side before you change to the other leg.

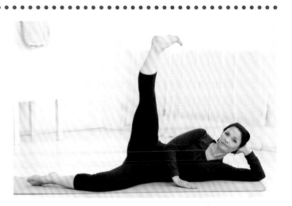

KNEE LIFTS (PAGE 101)

On your side, bend both legs and bring them forward to 90 degrees. Lift your upper leg up for 2 counts and down for 2 counts.
REPEAT 12 TIMES ON EACH SIDE.
Then lift your leg up and down for single counts, so this time a bit faster.

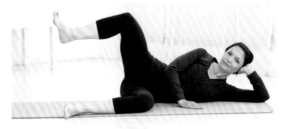

KICK KICK FORWARD
(PAGE 102)

Lie on your side and bring your lower leg
forward to 90 degrees. Flex your top foot and
kick forward in a 'one, two' beat at the end of
the kick to stetch the hamstring. Point your
toe as you return the leg and stretch through
the front of the thigh and hip flexor.
REPEAT 6 TIMES ON EACH SIDE.

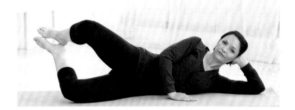

CLAMS (PAGE 103)

Lie on your side in a clam position, raise
your upper leg for a count of 2, then close
for a count of 2. **REPEAT 12 TIMES.**
On the last one, hold the clam open and
pulse for 12. **REPEAT ON THE OTHER SIDE.**

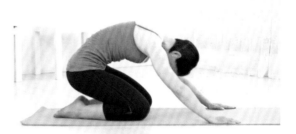

THE KITTY CAT (PAGE 122)

On all-fours, slowly curl your spine up and
then back, lowering your bottom before you
scoop down and forwards, and finally back up
to the start position. **REPEAT SLOWLY 6 TIMES.**

In the Zone:
5 Minute Arms

So, it's time to put the kettle on
and banish those bingo wings!

An exercise band is needed here.
Keep the band at a good tension
throughout to work your arms
hard. And move your neck gently
from side to side every so often
throughout this routine, to
prevent any discomfort.

LAT PULL DOWNS (PAGE 78)

Wrap the band around your hands. Begin with your arms above your head, palms facing forward and your feet hip-width apart, knees soft, with some weight in your heels. Breathe in, and as you exhale, connect and pull the band out to the sides, lowering it to the front of your chest while bringing the elbows down towards the ribcage. Your elbows should still be slightly bent at the bottom of the movement, and your wrists strong. Inhale as you return to the start position. **REPEAT 8 TIMES**.

Note – Try not to lose the tension in the band between repetitions.

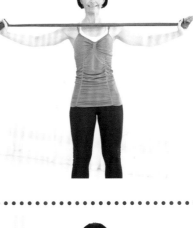

CHEST EXTENSIONS (PAGE 79)

From the same starting position as Lat Pull Downs, take the band behind your head. Breathe in, and as you exhale, connect and extend your elbows to lower the band down to your bottom. Keep the band close to your back as you go down. Inhale, and on the exhale, bend your elbows again to bring the band back up behind your head to the start position. **REPEAT 8 TIMES**.

Note – Try to keep your shoulders and arms moving evenly throughout this exercise.

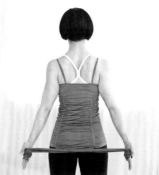

TRICEPS EXTENSIONS (PAGE 80)

Start in the same position as for Lat Pull Downs, but release a little tension in the band. Take your left hand behind your back, placing the back of your hand against your waist. Holding on to the band, and taking care to stand tall, bend your right arm over your head. Breathe in, and as you exhale, connect and straighten your right arm upwards, keeping your upper arm glued to the side of your head. Come back to the start position on the inhale. **REPEAT 8 TIMES ON EACH SIDE, MAINTAINING THE TENSION IN THE BAND.**

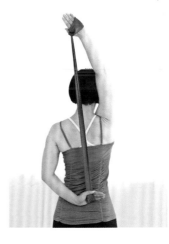

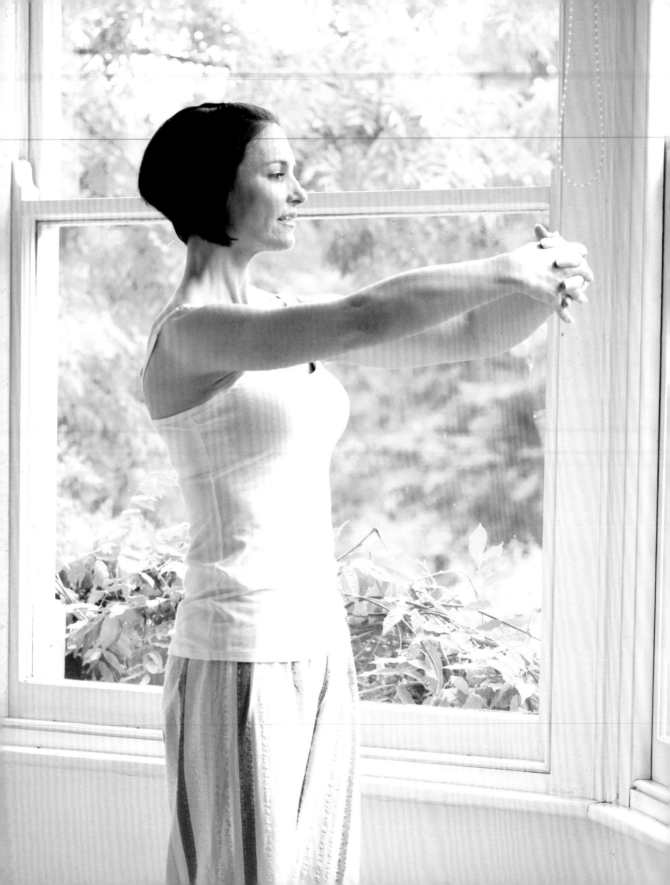

Life
on the go

One of the best things about Pilates and the other exercises I teach in my classes is that you can work so many of the Pilates principles into your daily life, boosting your general sense of health and wellbeing while keeping your fitness levels topped up at the same time. Furthermore, performed slowly, with precision, Pilates is a particularly calming form of exercise, which also really challenges your body. So it can be very beneficial in helping you to cope with the stresses and strains present in all our lives. I encourage all my clients to find a few moments in the day when they can relax, breathe and recharge, but I also encourage them to find some time to be active and get moving, from speed-walking with the baby buggy to doing a few bottom-toning squats and lunges before that latte and biscuit!

Working out doesn't necessarily mean having to find a full hour all in one go. You can exercise in short bursts between your other daily activities, or better still, combine exercising with your daily routine, for example by riding a bike to work or walking the children to school. On page 177 there are specific ideas for how to incorporate some fitness into your work day but here are just a few cardio boosting and toning activities to get you started.

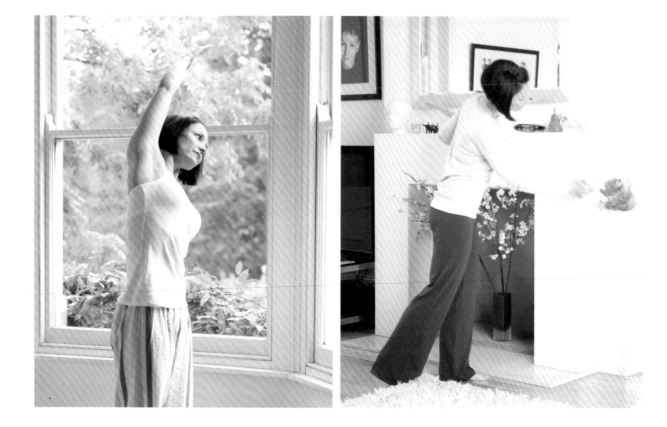

Exercise on the go

✳ Dancing is great exercise, so put on your favourite track and have a bop while doing the housework. When did you last dance around the house?

✳ Try various aerobic and dance/fitness classes. Figure out which ones work for you and try to schedule some time to go along each week. These will add variety to your week and keep your workouts fun and interesting; plus you'll meet other people who are also trying to get in shape.

✳ Massage your feet by rolling on a small ball while brushing your teeth – now this is an easy one and it feels wonderful!

✳ Stretch your hamstrings with a band while watching TV.

✳ Do your workouts during breaks in your favourite TV programme – Abs during the first intermission, Squats in the next one, then Lunges, Press-ups, arms with the band, Star Jumps, 30 seconds Skipping. You choose – it all adds up.

✳ Take the stairs two at a time.

✳ Practise your navel-to-spine connection – 30%, 60% and 100% – while sitting in traffic.

✳ Remember the pelvic floor? Work on it while on the phone, even to your bank manager. The person at the other end will never know!

✳ In the park, run from tree to tree, doing Star Jumps in-between, Press-ups at the next, and then some Skipping.

✳ Instead of going to the first sandwich shop at lunch time, walk briskly to one farther away.

✳ Sign up for a sponsored walk or run.

✳ 12 Press-ups against the back of your bedroom door – don't allow yourself to go through the doorway until you've done them.

✳ 20 Squat Jumps while making dinner.

✳ Speed walk in the park with the baby buggy, stopping every so often to do some Lunges or Squats.

✳ Remember you can fit in the 5 Minute Workouts any time of the day, so get going!

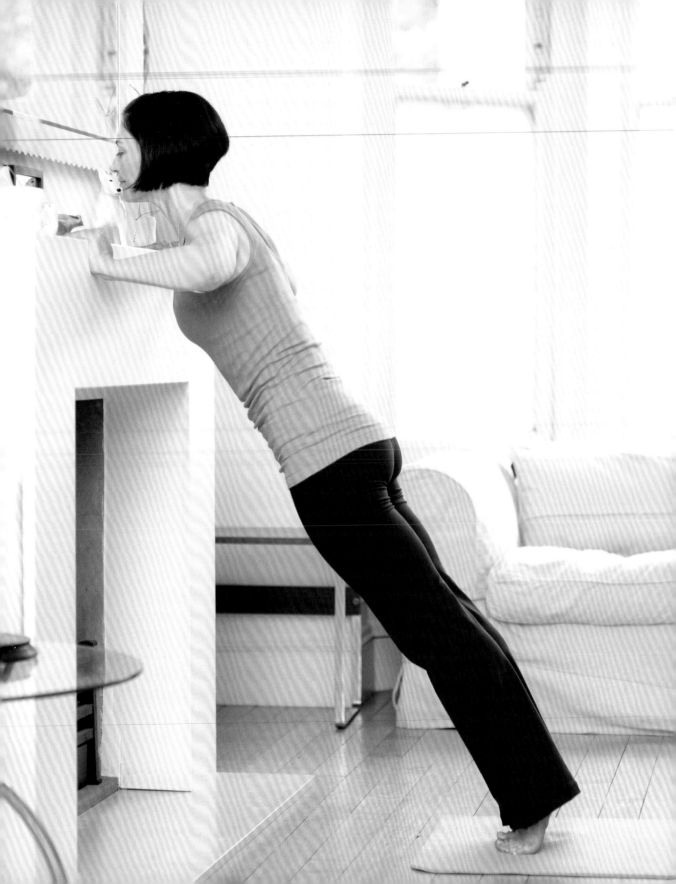

Home and Park Cardio Workouts

Whether the living room, garden or local park is the venue for your workout, you can use the following exercises to create a mini circuit. I've drawn up two on the following page, one for the home and the other for the park. These circuits work your whole body and improve your cardio fitness, but I've also designed them so that you can recover in-between each exercise. This means you can work at a high intensity, raising your heart rate and firing up your metabolism. Each circuit takes about 15 minutes, so don't be afraid to challenge yourself by increasing the time, distance or repetitions, or perhaps just go through the whole routine once more! Additionally, try incorporating light weights or a couple of water bottles into your home routine since these will help you burn more calories. But when the sun is shining, why not be outside? You can get in touch with nature and work out at the same time.

'After having my first baby I suffered from a split rectus abdominus, which didn't pull back together. I was advised by the physiotherapist to invest time and money in a good Pilates instructor as without it I was heading into a world of troubles. Margot worked me hard, tailoring everything very specifically to focus on reducing the gap. She taught me valuable lessons as to how to practise in between sessions in ways that I could fit into my daily life, walking around London pushing a buggy. Ten sessions later and the results were dramatic. The physiotherapist was thrilled and I could really see and feel the benefits. Almost a year on and I'm pregnant again and she is astonished at how small the bump is; she would have expected me to have burst already!' Hannah

Home Cardio

* 2 minutes of Jogging on the spot to warm you up
* 16 Lunges on each leg (use 2 light weights or water bottles if you want to work harder)
* 2 x 12 Standing Press-ups against a wall
* 30 seconds rest
* 30 High Knee Lifts on the spot
* 24 Step-ups on the stairs leading with the right leg, 24 leading with the left (using light weights/water bottles to challenge yourself)
* 100 Skips on the spot
* 30 seconds rest
* 30 Star Jumps
* 30 High Knee Lifts on the spot
* 3 x 12 seated Triceps Dips on the floor. Try lifting your bottom up 2 inch on the second set
* 30 seconds rest
* 100 Skips on the spot
* 12 Squats/12 Squats with a count of 2 at the bottom/12 Squat Jumps
* 30 High Knee Lifts on the spot
* 30 seconds rest
* 12 Burpees
* 100 Skips (with or without a skipping rope)
* Finish with 30 High Knee Lifts on the spot
* Stretch and a nice cup of tea!

Park Cardio

* One lap of the park – either Jogging or Speed Walking to warm you up
* Walking Lunges from one tree to the next (minimum 16)
* 2 x 12 Standing Press-ups against a tree or bench
* 30 seconds rest
* Run or Speed Walk to a park bench
* 12 Step-ups on to a bench leading with the right leg, 12 leading with the left
* Run or Speed Walk to the next tree
* 30 Star Jumps
* 30 seconds rest
* Run or Speed Walk to the next bench
* 3 x 12 Triceps Dips on the bench
* Run or Speed Walk to the next tree or bench
* 12 Squats/12 Squats with a count of 2 at the bottom/12 Squat Jumps
* 30 seconds rest
* Run or Speed Walk to the next tree
* 12 Burpees
* 100 Skips (with or without a skipping rope)
* Finish with 30 High Knee Lifts on the spot.
* Stretch and a nice low fat latte!

NOTE

– *Skipping: yes, I do mean get out that old skipping rope! If you don't have a skipping rope or the space to skip, imagine you do and perform the skips as if you are actually holding a skipping rope.*
– *If you do venture outside, take some time to enjoy the environment around you – perhaps linger for a post-exercise latte in the park. It will do wonders for your stress levels. This after-exercise reward may be all the encouragement you need to get you through your workout!*
– *Remember the sunscreen and some water, especially on warm days.*

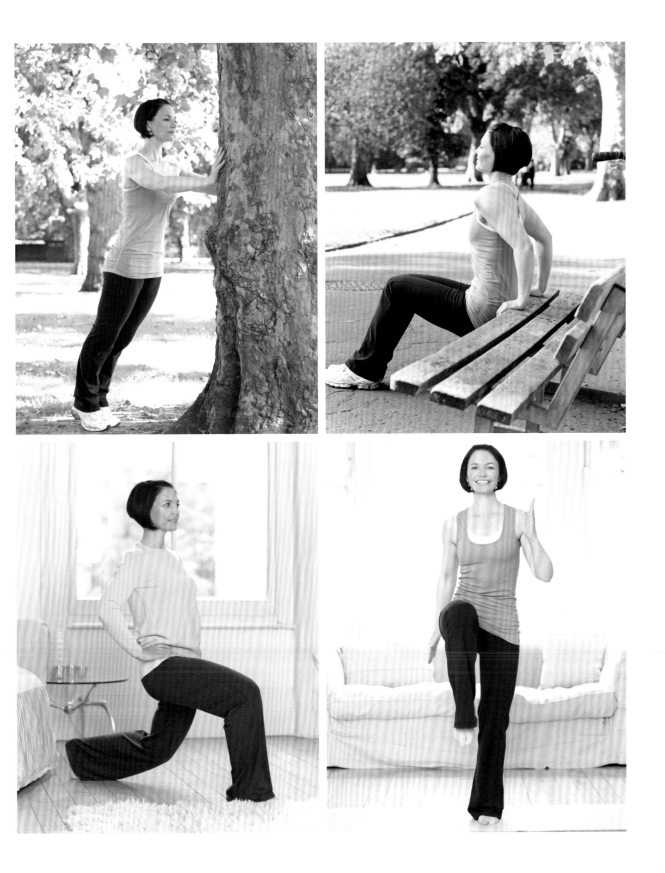

Home Cardio Workout

2 minutes of jogging on the spot to warm up

Come on… let's get going…

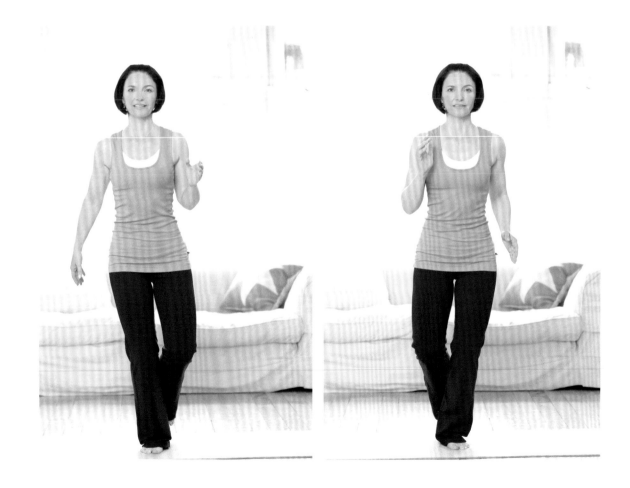

16 Lunges on each leg

1. Start with your feet hip-width apart, hands on hips.

2. Take a big step forward with your right leg, lifting your left heel so you are on the ball of your left foot. Keep your feet hip-width apart, like train tracks.

3. Breathe in, tuck your tailbone under and gently drop down.

Exhale, connect and push straight back up to the start position.

REPEAT 16 TIMES ON ONE LEG, THEN PULSE FOR 16 AT THE BOTTOM OF THE LAST LUNGE BEFORE SWAPPING TO THE OTHER LEG.

NOTE
– Make sure your front knee remains back behind your toe and your feet are hip-width apart. Check that your shoulders are directly above your hips and your back knee is directly below your hip.
– Make sure that you don't push forward while lunging, but perform a simple up and down motion using your bottom and legs.

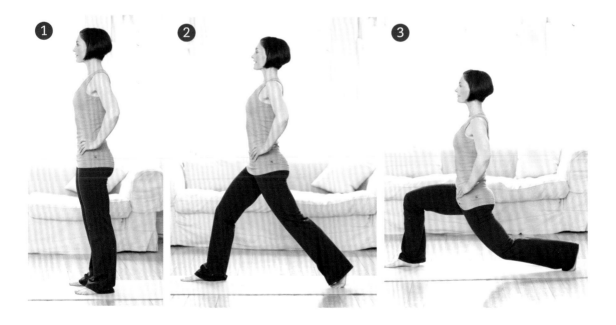

2 x 12 Standing Press-ups

1. Place your hands on the door or wall, slightly wider than shoulder-width apart but level with the shoulders. Your feet should be hip-width apart, your neck long (remember the triangle, page 73), your bottom down so that your body forms a straight diagonal line.

2. Inhale as you bend your arms to 90 degrees, or however close you can get while maintaining your line.

3. Exhale as you draw in your connection 100% and push back to the start position, pressing through the heel of your hands. Complete 2 sets of 12.

Then take 30 seconds rest.

NOTE

– For the challenging Triceps Press-up, position your hands below your shoulders, the elbows shaving the sides of your body as you perform the move.

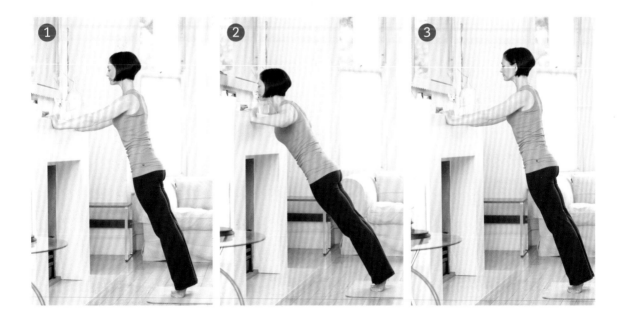

30 High Knee Lifts

Begin jogging on the spot, pumping your arms at the sides of your body as though you were running. Then gradually start to bring your knees up higher and faster.

Lift those knees...

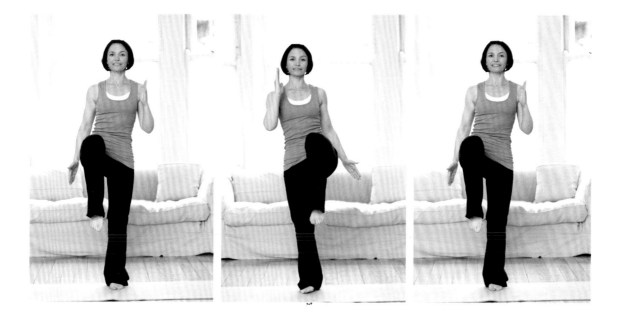

2 x 24 Step-ups on the stairs

1. Stand at the bottom of the stairs. Draw in your 60% navel-to-spine connection and breathe normally.

2. Step up on to the stair above with your right foot followed by your left. Then bring your right foot down followed by your left.

DO 24 STEP-UPS LEADING WITH THE RIGHT FOOT, AND ANOTHER 24 LEADING WITH THE LEFT FOOT.

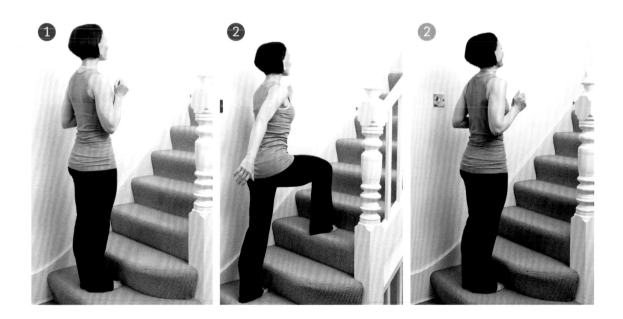

100 Skips (with or without a skipping rope)

If you don't have a skipping rope, just imagine you do. As you skip, be inventive and move from side to side, forward and back, even try some of the moves you remember from childhood, and then take 30 seconds rest.

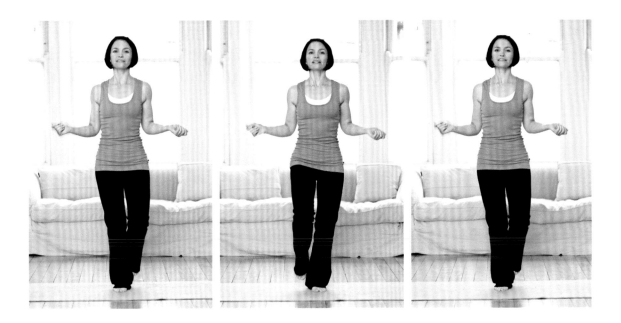

30 Star Jumps

1. Start with your feet together and your hands by your sides.

2. Breathe in. Exhale, connect and jump both feet out to the sides, raising your arms until your hands are just above shoulder height. Allow the inhale to happen naturally as you land and return your hands to your sides. Do 30 of these.

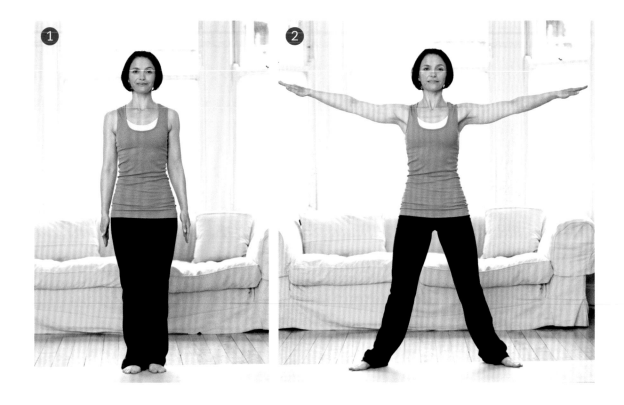

30 High Knee Lifts

Begin jogging on the spot, pumping your arms at the sides of your body as though you were running. Then gradually start to bring your knees up higher and faster.

You're halfway there...

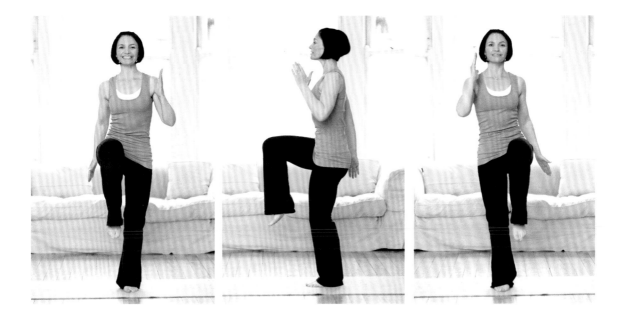

3 x 12 Triceps Dips

1. Sit on the floor, knees bent, feet together. Place your hands to the side of, and just behind your bottom, fingers facing forwards.

2. Breathe in as you bend your elbows back and lower your upper body towards the floor.

3. Exhale, connect and push back up to the start position, pressing through the palms of your hands and keeping your body straight, neck lengthened and relaxed. Complete 3 sets of 12 dips. Then take 30 seconds rest.

NOTE
– *To challenge yourself, lift your bottom 2 inches off the floor while performing the dips.*

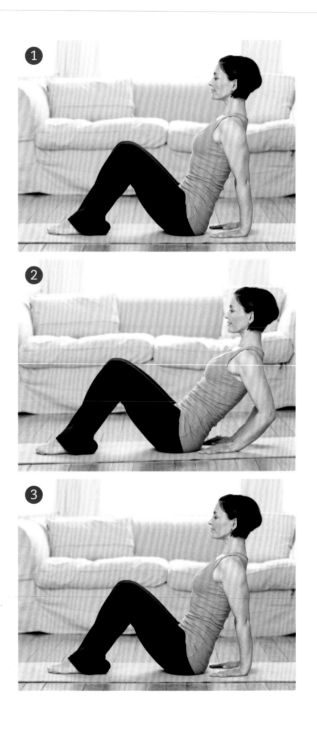

100 Skips (with or without a skipping rope)

If you don't have a skipping rope, just imagine you do. As you skip, be inventive and move from side to side, forward and back, even try some of the moves you remember from childhood, and then take 30 seconds rest.

Keep going...

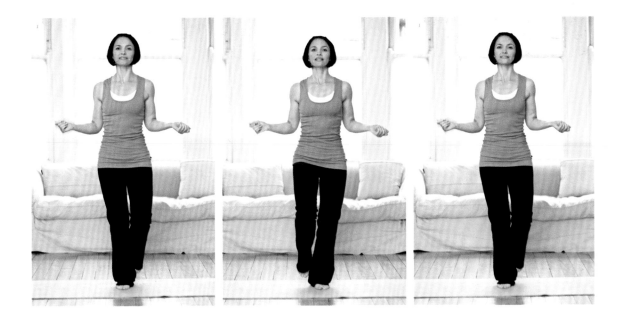

Squats

1. Stand with your feet hip-width apart, arms by your side.

2. Imagine you are going to sit back on to a chair. Breathe in as you squat down, keeping your back straight, arms extended and knees behind your toes. Exhale and connect as you push back up through your heels to the start position.

REPEAT 12 TIMES.

Now, squat down and hold the squat at the bottom for a count of 2 before pushing back up.

REPEAT 12 TIMES.

3. Finally, take your feet slightly wider and place your hands on your hips. Squat down and push through your toes as you explode back up to a standing position.

REPEAT 12 TIMES.

NOTE
– *Keep your shoulders relaxed and don't let your knees drift forward beyond your toes while performing the Squats.*
– *Remember to maintain your connection throughout to protect your lower back.*
– *If you experience discomfort in the lower back, don't squat so low. Also check that you are still drawing in your connection. Once you get the hang of the movement, you can always try deepening the Squat again.*

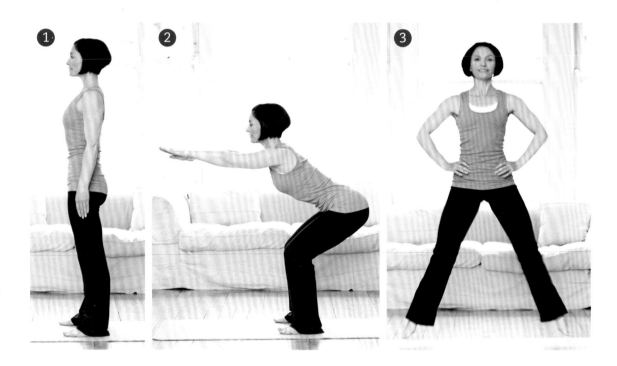

30 High Knee Lifts

Begin jogging on the spot, pumping your arms at the sides of your body as though you were running. Then gradually start to bring your knees up higher and faster.

Take 30 seconds rest.

Shall I put the coffee on?...

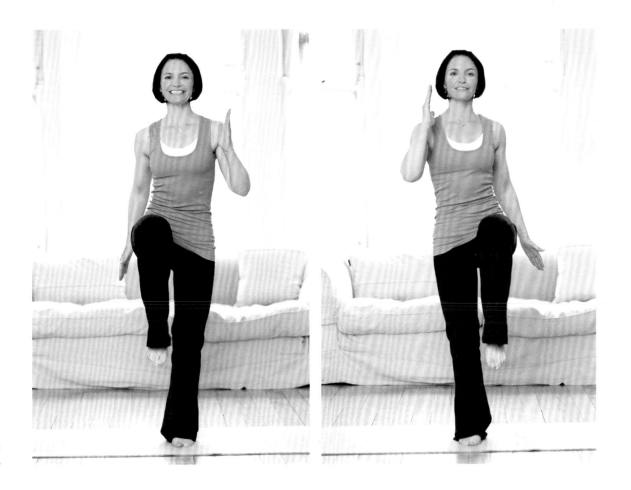

12 Burpees

1. Begin in a standing position and inhale as you drop into a crouched position with your hands on the ground beside your feet.

2. In one quick movement, exhale and connect as you jump and extend your legs straight out behind you so you are in the Full Press-up start position.

3. Inhale as you jump your feet back to the crouching position.

4. Exhale as you leap up to standing.

REPEAT 12 TIMES.

NOTE
– *If it is too difficult to jump both feet forward or back together, take them back one at a time to begin with.*

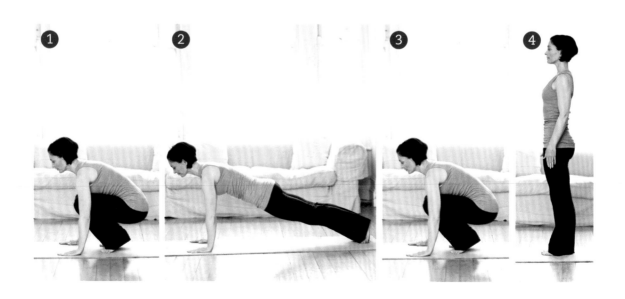

100 Skips

Nearly there...

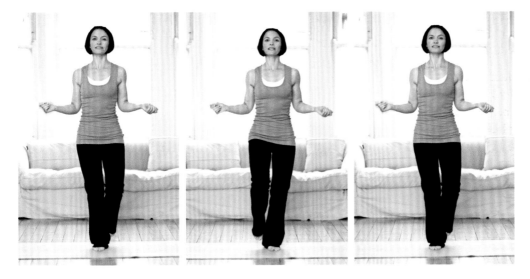

30 High Knee Lifts

You made it... well done!

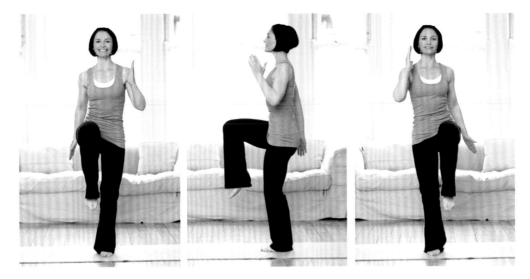

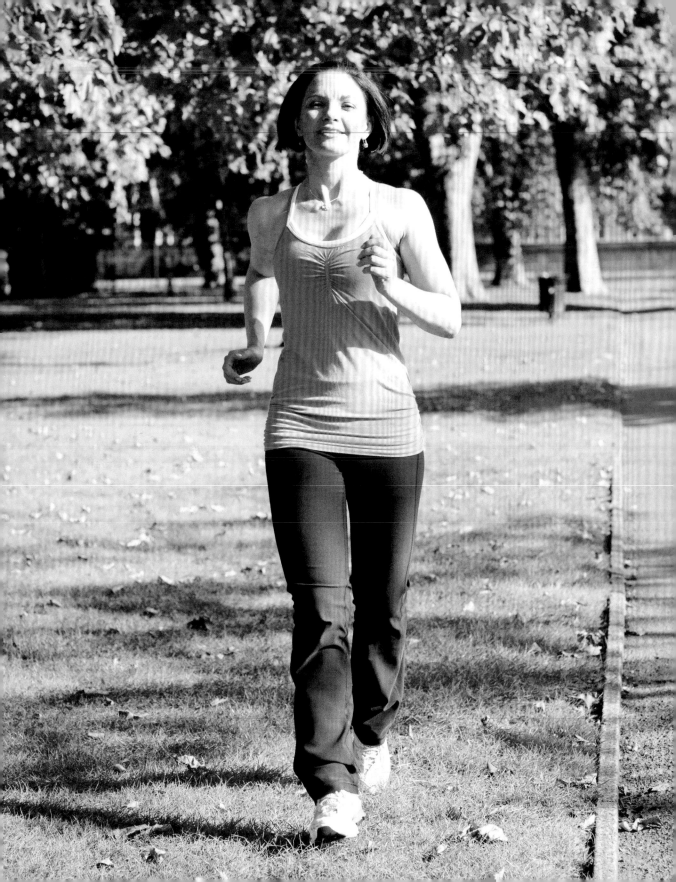

Park Cardio Workout

One lap of the park – either Jogging or Speed Walking to warm up

Whether you're running or speed walking, make sure you are going at a pace that is right for you. So, stand tall and pump your arms from your shoulders as you go.

Remember, this is your workout!

Walking Lunges from one tree to the next (minimum 16)

1. Start with your feet hip-width apart, hands on hips.

2. Take a big step forward with your right leg, lifting your left heel so you are on the ball of your left foot. Keep your feet hip-width apart, like train tracks.

3. Breathe in, tuck your tailbone under and gently drop down.

4. Exhale, connect, and push up from the back leg, stepping forward into the next lunge.

REPEAT AT LEAST 16 TIMES AS YOU LUNGE FROM ONE TREE TO THE NEXT.

NOTE
– *Make sure your front knee remains back behind your toe and your feet are hip-width apart. Check that your shoulders are directly above your hips and your back knee is directly below your hip.*
– *Make sure that you don't push your body forward while completing the Walking Lunges, but perform a simple up and down motion using your bottom and legs.*

2 x 12 Standing Press-ups against a tree or bench

1. Place your hands on the bench, slightly wider than shoulder-width apart. Your feet should be hip-width apart, your neck long (remember the triangle, page 73), your bottom down so that your body forms a straight diagonal line.

2. Inhale as you bend your arms to 90 degrees, or however close you can get while maintaining your line.

3. Exhale as you draw in your connection 100% and push back to the start position, pressing through the heel of your hands.

COMPLETE 2 SETS OF 12.

Then take 30 seconds rest.

Run or Speed Walk to a park bench

Come on... pick up the pace!

2 x 12 Step-ups on to a bench

1. Stand about a foot away from the bench. Draw in your 60% navel-to-spine connection and breathe normally.

2. Step up on to the bench with your right foot followed by your left. Then bring your right foot down followed by your left.
DO 12 STEP-UPS LEADING WITH THE RIGHT FOOT, AND ANOTHER 12 LEADING WITH THE LEFT FOOT.

Run or Speed Walk to the next tree

You're halfway...

Excellent... keep moving...

30 Star Jumps

1. Start with your feet together and your hands by your sides.

2. Breathe in. Exhale, connect and jump both feet out to the sides, raising your arms until your hands are just above shoulder height. Allow the inhale to happen naturally as you land and return your hands to your sides.
REPEAT 30 TIMES.

Take 30 seconds rest.

Run or Speed Walk to the next bench

You're halfway...

3 x 12 Triceps Dips on bench

1. Position your bottom near the edge of the bench, your hands on either side, fingers facing forwards.

2. Keep your head up and breathe in as you slowly lower your body down until your elbows are at right angles facing backwards.

3. As you exhale, connect and push back up to the start position.
COMPLETE 3 SETS OF 12 DIPS.

NOTE
– *The farther away your feet are from the bench, the harder the exercise will be, so begin by moving your feet away just a little and then increase the distance as you become stronger and more familiar with the exercise.*
– *Be careful to take your elbows back as you dip down; they shouldn't go out to the sides at all.*

Run or Speed Walk to the next tree or bench

You're doing so well, so keep going... that coffee is just around the corner!

12 Squats/12 Squats with a count of 2 at the bottom/12 Squat Jumps

1. Stand with your feet hip-width apart, arms by your side.

2. Imagine you are going to sit back on to a chair. Breathe in as you squat down, keeping your back straight, arms extended and knees behind your toes.

3. Exhale and connect as you push back up through your heels to the start position.
REPEAT 12 TIMES.

4. Now, squat down and hold the squat at the bottom for a count of 2 before pushing back up.
REPEAT 12 TIMES.

5. Finally, take your feet slightly wider and place your hands on your hips. Squat down and push through your toes as you explode back up to a standing position. **REPEAT 12 TIMES.**

Take 30 seconds rest.

NOTE
– Keep your shoulders relaxed and don't let your knees drift forward beyond your toes while performing the squats.
– Remember to maintain your connection throughout to protect your lower back.
– If you experience discomfort in the lower back muscles, don't squat so low. Also check that you are still drawing in your connection. Once you get the hang of the movement, you can always try deepening the squat again.

*Run or Speed Walk
to the next tree*

You must be able
to smell the coffee
by now!

12 Burpees

1. Begin in a standing position and inhale as you drop into a crouched position with your hands on the ground beside your feet.

2. In one quick movement, exhale and connect as you jump and extend your legs straight out behind you so you are in the Full Press-up start position.

3. Inhale as you jump your feet back to the crouching position.

4. Exhale as you leap up to standing.
REPEAT 12 TIMES.

NOTE
– If it is too difficult to jump both feet forward or back together, take them back one at a time to begin with.

100 Skips (with or without a skipping rope)

If you don't have a skipping rope, just imagine you do. As you skip, be inventive and move from side to side, forward and back, even try some of the moves you remember from childhood!

30 High Knee Lifts

Begin jogging on the spot, pumping your arms at the sides of your body as though you were running. Then gradually start to bring your knees up higher and faster.

You made it...
well done!

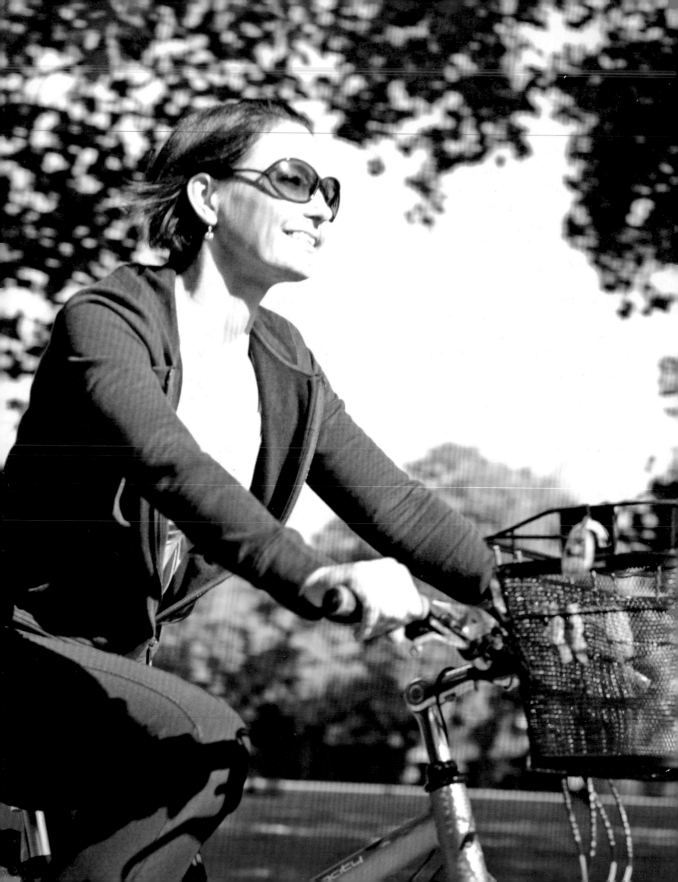

Working 9–5

Many of us spend a good deal of our day at work, perhaps sitting behind a desk or standing for long periods of time. Whether sitting or standing, remember to think tall (30% connection) as though a thread is gently pulling you up from the very top of your head. So why not try going through your day being more aware of your body, and consider some of the ideas below on how to keep yourself more active. An active body encourages an active and focused mind.

✳ Take the stairs instead of the lift.

✳ Go and talk to someone rather than sending an email.

✳ Instead of bringing a full bottle of water to your desk every morning, go and fetch a glass of water whenever you need one.

✳ Use toilet facilities on another floor.

✳ Go for a walk or a run at lunchtime and get some fresh air.

✳ Practise your pelvic floor exercises at your desk, sitting on the bus, pretty much anywhere. That includes some bottom clenching!

✳ Get off the bus/tube early and walk some of the way.

✳ Practise drawing in your navel towards your spine first to 30%, then 60% and finally 100%.

✳ For a burst of energy, do 20 step-ups on the stairs, or just climb a few more floors!

✳ Try cycling to work or the railway station to wake you up first thing in the morning!

How to set up your work space

We were born to move, so if you spend a great deal of time sitting at a desk, make sure you get up and walk around every half-hour or so whenever possible. Sitting for too long increases stiffness, back pain, neck and shoulder problems, headaches, eye strain and repetitive strain injuries, and often gives us a general feeling of agitation, or sometimes lethargy and a lack of energy. So it's good to get your energy flowing every now and then.

Check your desk is set up correctly, which basically means in a way that won't have you acting like a contortionist every time you go to answer the phone.

* Start by getting an adjustable chair, so that the chair swivels rather than you having to twist, and learn how to use it! Adjust the height so that your wrists are resting comfortably on the desk just in front of your keyboard. Your feet should be flat on the floor. If they're not, get a footrest or improvise (a lever arch file is perfect!). Arm rests should be adjusted so that your elbows can rest on them without causing discomfort in the shoulders (you may need to position the arm rests slightly lower than the desk). The back rest should give you adequate support, but place a small cushion at the base of your spine if necessary.

* Position your computer screen about an arm's length away from you, eyes level with the top of the screen. Slightly tilt the screen to reduce any glare. Pushing the screen too far back will result in you sitting forward in your chair, straining to see what's displayed on it. You will also probably feel some discomfort in the back since nothing will be supporting it.

* Check that the keyboard is right in front of you and your upper body is not slightly twisted to one side when using it. Try positioning the keyboard slightly to the right if you don't use the number pad, preventing any twisting in the body.

* Check that your mouse hasn't wandered off up the desk during the day as you've changed position, causing you to overstretch to reach it and creating discomfort in the shoulder area.

* Attach a document holder to the side of the screen if you do a lot of typing and looking at documents at the same time. This will help prevent any discomfort in your neck and upper body.

* If you are on the phone frequently, use a headset rather than holding the receiver for long periods of time. This also lets you type or write easily at the same time, rather than twisting your body uncomfortably. If you don't use a headset, position the phone so that you can very easily reach it with your non-writing hand.

* Keep your desk and the area below it clear of clutter so that everything you need is easily accessible, and you don't feel hemmed in at all, which can create stress in your body.

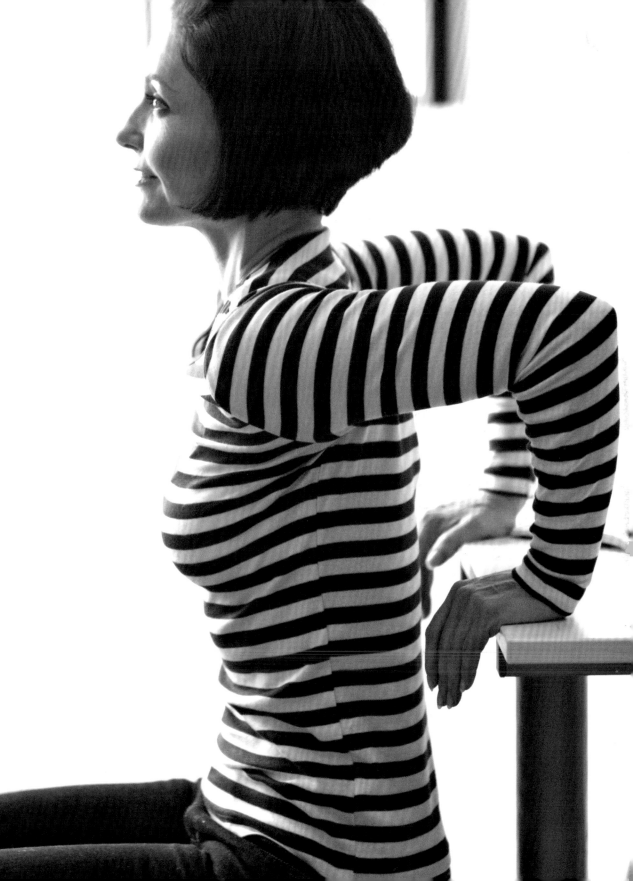

The desk workout

I've devised a mini series of stretches and exercises for the times you are desk-bound. Do a few of these during the day and you'll prevent stiffness or tension setting in. They are a great wake-up for your brain too, if you spend long periods of the day concentrating or looking at a computer screen. Remember to try to get up and move around every 30 minutes, rather than remaining stuck in the same position for hours on end.

Neck Releases

1. Sitting up with 30% navel-to-spine connection, take one hand up over your head so it just touches the top of your opposite ear. Gently press your head to the side, towards your upraised arm, breathing in to the side of the neck you are stretching.

HOLD THIS FOR 3 BREATHS IN AND OUT AND THEN SWAP OVER TO THE OTHER SIDE.

2. Now take your hand up and over the top of your head and look towards your armpit as you stretch the back of the neck. Imagine breathing in to the part of your neck that is stretching.

HOLD THIS FOR 3 BREATHS IN AND OUT THEN REPEAT ON THE OTHER SIDE.

3. Facing forward, bring both hands up together, resting them on the crown of the head, keeping your elbows as close as you can, and gently press your head forward, feeling and breathing into the back of the neck.

DO THIS FOR 3 BREATHS IN AND OUT.

4. Now draw in your navel-to-spine connection 60% and continue to press your head forward gently as you also curl your spine to stretch the back.

DO THIS FOR 3 BREATHS IN AND OUT.

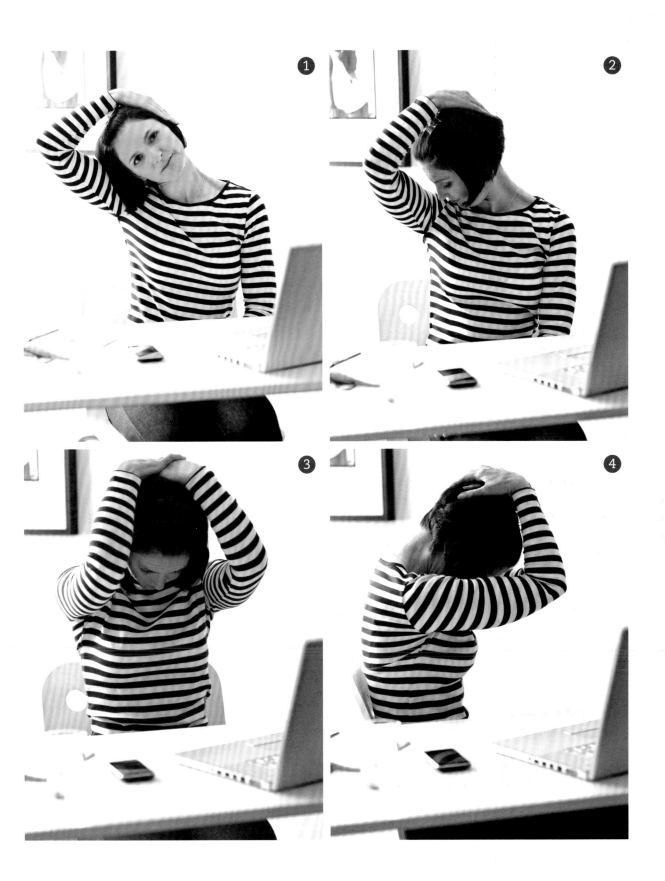

Upper Body Strengthening

PRESS-UPS AGAINST A DESK
(PAGE 160)

Place hands slightly wider than shoulder-width apart on a desk or wall, feet hip-width apart, your neck long, and your bottom down forming a straight diagonal line. Inhale as you bend your arms to 90 degrees. Exhale as you draw in your connection 100% and push back to the start position, pressing through the heel of your hands.

COMPLETE 2 SETS OF 12.

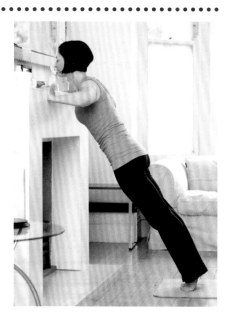

TRICEPS DIPS (PAGE 166)

Position yourself at the edge of your desk, hands to the sides of your bottom, fingers facing forwards. Draw in your connection. Breathe in as you bend your elbows back and lower your upper body towards the floor. Push back up to the start position as you exhale, pressing through the palms of your hands and keeping your body straight, neck lengthened and relaxed.

COMPLETE 2 SETS OF 8 DIPS.

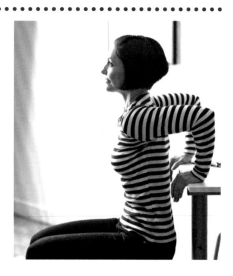

Ankle Mobility

• •

ANKLE ROTATIONS

Rotate each ankle 3 times in each direction with your toes pointed. Then repeat with your toes flexed.

Lower Body Conditioning

• •

SQUATS (PAGE 106)

Breathe in as you squat down until you just touch your chair, exhale and connect as you push back up through your heels. **REPEAT 12 TIMES**.

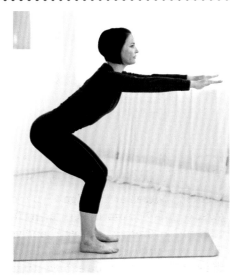

Upper Body Stretches

UPPER BACK STRETCH (PAGE 91)

Sit with arms out in front of you, fingers clasped together. As you exhale, connect and gently push your hands away from the body. Hold for a few seconds before release.
REPEAT 3 TIMES.

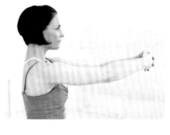

TRICEPS STRETCH (PAGE 90)

Take your right arm up behind your head, placing the palm of your hand in between your shoulder blades. Take your left arm up and over to grasp the right elbow. As you exhale, connect and press down on the elbow to stretch the back of the arm. Hold for a few seconds before release.
REPEAT 3 TIMES ON EACH SIDE.

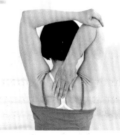

SHOULDER STRETCH (PAGE 90)

Sit with right arm stretched straight across your body, palm open. Place your left hand on your right upper arm. As you exhale, connect and draw the right arm towards you. Hold for a few seconds before release.
REPEAT 3 TIMES ON EACH SIDE.

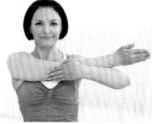

CHEST STRETCH (PAGE 91)

Sit with hands clasped behind your back while keeping your neck and shoulders relaxed and your back straight. Exhale, connect and lift your arms out behind you until you feel the stretch across the chest. Hold for a few seconds before release. **REPEAT 3 TIMES.**

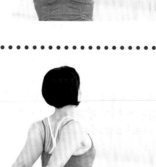

Arm Band Exercises

LAT PULL DOWNS (PAGE 78)

Begin with the band wrapped around your hands, arms above your head, palms forward, feet hip-width apart. As you exhale, connect and pull the band out to the sides, lowering it to the front of your chest while bringing the elbows down towards the ribcage. Your elbows should still be slightly bent at the bottom of the movement, and your wrists strong. Inhale as you return to the start position. **REPEAT 8 TIMES.**

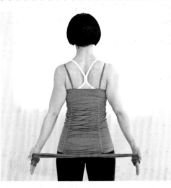

CHEST EXTENSIONS (PAGE 79)

From the same starting position as Lat Pull Downs, take the band behind your head. As you exhale, connect and extend your elbows to lower the band down to your bottom. Keep the band close to your back as you go down. Inhale, and on the exhale, bend your elbows again to bring the band back up behind your head to the start position. **REPEAT 8 TIMES.**

TRICEPS EXTENSIONS (PAGE 80)

Start in the same position as for Lat Pull Downs, but with less tension in the band. Take your left hand behind your back, placing the back of your hand against your waist. Bend your right arm over your head. As you exhale, connect and straighten your right arm upwards, keeping your upper arm glued to the side of your head. Come back to the start position on the inhale. **REPEAT 8 TIMES ON EACH SIDE, MAINTAINING THE TENSION IN THE BAND.**

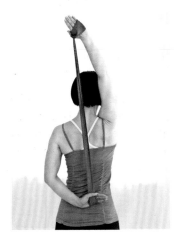

Stress busting

Most of us live such busy lives nowadays it's no wonder we tend to feel a bit overwhelmed by stress every now and again. Healthy living is a fantastic way to prevent stress from building up, and it also gives us helpful ways to relieve stress when it does hit hard. This is why I encourage all my clients to add healthy habits to their daily lives, rather than going on a blitz detox and fitness regime for just a few intense days at a time and reverting to their sometimes less healthy, sedentary lives for the rest of the time. Little and often pays huge dividends when it comes to coping really well with the stresses and strains of modern life.

In a stressful situation, the body goes into 'fight or flight' mode. We produce a burst of adrenalin so that we can react superfast – either getting away from danger or standing and fighting. This was really helpful when human beings spent their lives in the wild, but now that we don't often need to fight or flee in a stressful situation, all that adrenalin has nowhere to go and we end up feeling stressed-out with our nerves on edge.

A little stress in our lives is actually a good thing because it keeps us on our toes and gives us a bit of get up and go. However, if stress levels stay too high for too long, we start to feel the effects of adrenal burnout. Our energy deserts us. Many people find it hard to get to sleep at night as their minds buzz with worries or the endless 'things to do' list. And then it's equally hard to get up in the morning, let alone jump out of bed with a spring in your step!

One of the reasons I took up Pilates was because at the time I was a very busy person, always rushing from one place to another, cramming in so much that I was starting to feel as though there weren't enough hours in the day and my stress levels weren't getting an adequate chance to recover. For me, discovering that Pilates could be a flowing and calming form of exercise but could also work your body really hard made it irresistible. I have never looked back. Now I practise most days, combining many of the strength, stretching and breathing aspects to recharge my body and give me a balanced approach to my exercise and lifestyle.

Physically, stress is often felt in the shoulders, neck and back, and so gentle exercises that work on these areas of the body can be great allies in the battle against the stresses and strains of modern living. Try the neck-release exercises on page 180 and the upper body stretches on pages 90-91, or have a go at the breathing and stretching exercises in the warm-up and cool-down routines. These are all designed to help stretch and lengthen the body and relieve discomfort.

Workout to work things out

So how exactly does exercise help to keep our stress levels in a healthy balance?

✶ Exercise releases 'feel good' hormones called endorphins, which give the body a natural, relaxed high.

✶ Concentrating on your body while exercising takes your mind off everything else, giving you a welcome distraction from any worries.

✶ A good workout provides a physical release for any negative emotions that have been bubbling up throughout the day.

✶ Taking care of your body has been shown to boost confidence and self-esteem, so you are less likely to let stress get the better of you.

✶ Being more aware of your body means you spot the signs of stress earlier, so you can take preventive action before it has a chance to set in.

'I was a complete stress head before I took up Pilates. I worked all hours and never devoted any time to myself, although I had a nagging feeling that if I could just take care of my fitness a bit more I would feel better about everything. Since taking up Pilates I have become so much calmer. It's like a meditation for me but I am also toning and shaping my body like never before. Just a couple of hours a week and suddenly I feel like I'm better equipped to tackle my stressful day. Looking after your body definitely helps look after your mind.' Helen

Calm and collected

Many of my clients lead superbusy and stressful lives and over time I have discovered some great natural stress relievers.

Relaxation visualisation

Take a minute to bring to mind a completely relaxing image or experience. It may be walking along your favourite beach, the sand beneath your toes, the sound and feel of the waves gently rolling in and out with the tide; or you might imagine a person who makes you feel calm and relaxed. If you ever feel negative emotions or stress bubbling up inside you so much that you feel you may burst, sit quietly and transport yourself to your favourite relaxing place or into the company of your calming friend. Then try some lateral breathing (page 45) slowly and deeply for a few minutes.

Breathe

Controlling your breathing is essential for Pilates and, for me, unites body and mind. When stressed, you might find yourself breathing in a shallower, less efficient way. Your body tenses up from your shoulders to your neck to your tummy, and so your breathing also becomes more tense, depriving your body of vital and relaxing oxygen. Try becoming more aware of your breathing, and if need be, take a couple of really mindful breaths, slow and deep at first and then at a natural pace. This has an immediate calming effect that money just can't buy.

Rest well

A good workout will tire you out physically and is often mentally calming, helping you to sleep like a proverbial baby. A warm aromatherapy bath or shower in the evening will help your muscles to recover and will also gently help you to relax before going to bed. After your bath, do some gentle stretches and steer clear of your computer or electronic gadgets for at least a couple of hours before you go to sleep to give your mind a chance to slow down and unwind. If you keep your afternoon and evening caffeine free and drink herbal teas, such as peppermint and chamomile, instead, you'll have a good chance of nodding off quickly for a night of energising, revitalising sleep.

If you wake up in the morning feeling stiff and sore and worse than you did before you went to bed, try sleeping on your side in the foetal position – shoulder on top of shoulder, hip on top of hip, knee on top of knee, with the feet either together or slightly split. The head should be aligned with the rest of the spine and supported by a comfortable pillow. This position may not be the most comfortable to begin with but try it for a few weeks and see if this makes a difference to how your body feels in the morning!

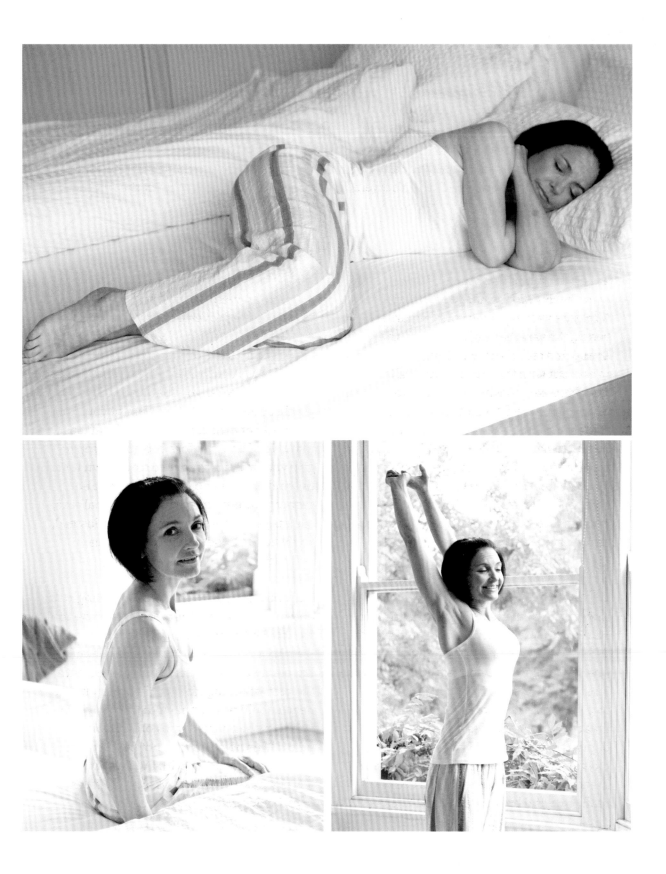

It has given me great pleasure this summer to spend time sharing my ideas with you on how to balance and combine exercise with today's busy lifestyles. So I hope you find they work for you like they have done for so many of my clients and that you too recognise that a balance of Pilates and everyday fitness activities is a wonderful way of exercising and achieving the body you've always been looking for!

Margot x

www.pilatesonthego.co.uk

Acknowledgements

No task is ever accomplished alone so I'd especially like to thank all my clients and friends who have contributed and encouraged me throughout this project, especially Anne, Rhi, Emma, Patricia, Sally, Suellen, Aileen, Sonia, Caroline, Bridget, Amanda and Clare.

I'd also like to thank Kate for her advice and support throughout and my agent Diana, together with Nicky and Sarah at Hodder & Stoughton and Emma at Smith & Gilmour.

Finally, thank you to all those at Jet Studios, Sarah for her styling and tweaking, Jo for my hair and make-up and Sweaty Betty for my wardrobe.

First published in Great Britain in 2012
by Hodder & Stoughton
An Hachette UK company

1

Copyright © Margot Campbell 2012

The right of Margot Campbell to be identified as the Author of the Work has been asserted by her in accordance with the Copyright, Designs and Patents Act 1988.

A CIP catalogue record for this title is available from the British Library.

Trade Paperback ISBN 978 1 444 73890 2
Ebook ISBN 978 1 444 73891 9

Designed and typeset in
PMN Caecillia by Smith & Gilmour

Printed and bound in the UK by Butler Tanner & Dennis Ltd

Hodder & Stoughton policy is to use papers that are natural, renewable and recyclable products and made from wood grown in sustainable forests. The logging and manufacturing processes are expected to conform to the environmental regulations of the country of origin.

Hodder & Stoughton Ltd
338 Euston Road
London NW1 3BH
www.hodder.co.uk

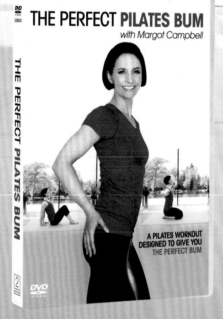
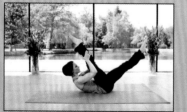
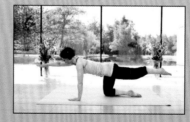
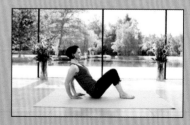